The Future of Mental Health Services: Coping with Crisis

Leonard J. Duhl, M.D., is Professor of Public Health and City and Regional Planning at the University of California, Berkeley, with an additional teaching appointment in psychiatry at the University of California, San Francisco Medical Center.

His extensive publications include *The Urban Condition* (1963), which concerns the quality of life in cities and their relationship to health, and the recently published *Healthy Social Change*, a compilation of his writings over the years.

His work has included evaluating the relative "health" of cities in the United States, Canada, China, and recently, in Europe as consultant for the World Health Organization.

Nicholas A. Cummings, Ph.D. was Senior Psychologist with the Kaiser Permanente Health System for 25 years. He is a past president of the American Psychological Association (1979–1980) and the founding President of the four campuses of the California School of Professional Psychology. He is currently the President of the Biodyne Institute and the President and C.E.O. of the American Biodyne Centers, Inc. He is also the President, in Washington, DC, of the nine National Academies of Practice, limited to 100 distinguished practitioners in each profession of dentistry, medicine, optometry, osteopathic medicine, podiatric medicine, psychology, social work, and veterinary medicine.

The Future of Mental Health Services:
Coping with Crisis

Leonard J. Duhl, M.D.
Nicholas A. Cummings, Ph.D.
Editors

with the assistance of
James J. Hynes, M.P.H., M.C.P.

SPRINGER PUBLISHING COMPANY
New York

Springer Publishing Company, Inc.
536 Broadway
New York, NY 10012

87 88 89 90 91 / 5 4 3 2 1

Library of Congress Cataloging-in-Publication Data

The Future of mental health services.

   Includes bibliographies and index.
   1. Mental health services—Unites States.
I. Duhl, Leonard J. II. Cummings, Nicholas A.
[DNLM: 1. Mental Health Services—trends—United
States. WM 30 F996]
RA790.6.F88   1986   362.2'0973   86-28030
ISBN 0-8261-5840-4

Printed in the United States of America

Contents

Contributors

Robert A. Aldrich, M.D., has a long and distinguished career in health services, particularly in the areas of child health, human ecology, urbanization, health policy, education and training of health professionals, and health services planning and administration. Among other honors, he has been named a Distinguished Fellow of the American Psychiatric Association and has received the E. Mead Johnson Award for Pediatric Research. He is currently Clinical Professor in the Department of Pediatrics at the University of Washington.

Ralph A. Catalano, Ph.D., is Professor of Social Ecology and Management at the University of California, Irvine. He is also Assistant Vice Chancellor for Plans and Programs and serves as a member of the Irvine City Council. He holds a Ph.D. in social science from Syracuse University. His research into the mental health effects of economic perturbation is described in several of the articles cited in the chapter he has prepared for this volume.

Luther P. Christman, Ph.D., R.N., holds degrees in nursing, clinical psychology, and sociology and anthropology. He is currently the John L. and Helen Kellogg Dean, College of Nursing, Rush University, and Vice President for Nursing Affairs, Rush-Presbyterian-St. Luke's Medical Center, Chicago. He is the recipient of numerous awards and honors, notably the Edith Moore Copeland Founder's Award for Creativity, Sigma Theta Tau, and honorary membership in Alpha Omega Alpha, the honor society of medicine.

Burr Eichelman, M.D., Ph.D. is Professor of Psychiatry at the University of Wisconsin-Madison and Chief of Psychiatry at the William S. Middleton Memorial VA Hospital. He received his

M.D. and Ph.D. (in biopsychology) from the University of Chicago and received residency training in psychiatry at Stanford University. He spent one year as a Kennedy Fellow in Medicine, Law and Ethics.

Saul Feldman, Ph.D., is currently president of General Parametrics Corporation and of the Bay Area Foundation for Human Services in Berkeley, CA. He was formerly president of Health America Corporation of California and executive director of the Rockridge Health Care Plan. Earlier at the National Institute of Mental Health he served as director of the Staff College and of the Community Mental Health Centers program.

Dr. Feldman has published widely on health administration and community mental health. He is the founder and editor of the journal *Administration of Mental Health* and former president of the American College in Mental Health Administration. His academic affiliations include an appointment as faculty associate in the School of Public Health at the Johns Hopkins University; visiting Professor of Psychiatry and behavioral sciences at the State University of New York at Stony Brook; adjunct Professor of Psychiatry at the Uniformed Services University of the Health Sciences; and visiting lecturer at the University of Southern California.

Shervert H. Frazier, M.D., is Director of the National Institute of Mental Health (NIMH), a component of the U.S. Department of Health and Human Services Alcohol, Drug Abuse, and Mental Health Administration. Before assuming this position in 1984, he was Psychiatrist-in-Chief of McLean Hospital and Professor of Psychiatry, Harvard Medical School. He has held senior faculty and administrative positions with the Department of Psychiatry, Columbia University College of Physicians and Surgeons/New York State Psychiatric Institute and the Baylor University School of Medicine, and has served as Commissioner of Mental Health and Mental Retardation for the State of Texas.

Timothy J. Gallagher, M.A., has been the Director of Admissions and Financial Aid for the four campuses of the California School of Professional Psychology since 1980. Prior to that he was the Admissions Officer in the Central Administration of the School for two and one-half years. In his role directing the marketing of CSPP, he has spent much time researching current trends, and frequently gives informational lectures about the future of the mental health profession at colleges and universities. His academic background includes training at the baccalaureate and masters level in philosophy from the University of Santa Clara and University of California at Berkeley, respectively.

Beth Goldman, M.D., M.P.H. is completing a Residency in Psychiatry at the Langley Porter Psychiatric Institute, University of California, San Francisco. She received her M.P.H. from Yale University in 1976 and worked as an epidemiologist at the Center for Disease Control, Venereal Disease Control Division, until entering the University of Michigan Medical School in 1978. She has just completed an innovative interactive computer program designed to teach beginning medical students how to diagnose and treat psychiatric disorders. She has publications in the *Journal of the American College Health Association*, the *Journal of the American Public Health Association* and with the Upjohn Company, and she has presented papers before the American Public Health Association.

Anne Hartwig, Ph.D., J.D., is currently Senior Council in the Department of Public Instruction for the State of Wisconsin and a lecturer at the University of Wisconsin-Madison. She received her J.D. and Ph.D. (in Educational Administration) at the University of Wisconsin.

James J. Hynes, M.P.H., M.C.P. received his BA from the State University of New York at Stony Brook in 1980 and his duel Masters in Public Health and City Planning in 1985. He now works as a program evaluator for the Yolo Community Care Continuum in Davis, California and as a research associate at the Institute for Health Policy Studies, School of Medicine, University of California at San Francisco. He has recently begun work on a book about cities and health.

Charles A. Kiesler, Ph.D., is Provost and Professor of Psychology at Vanderbilt University, Nashville, Tennessee. He previously held positions as Walter Van Dyke Bingham Professor of Psychology and Dean of the College of Humanities and Social Sciences at Carnegie-Mellon University. Prior to that, he was Executive Officer of the American Psychological Association. He received his Ph.D. from Stanford University and was formerly Chair of the Ph.D. Program in Personality and Social Psychology at Yale University. He has published numerous articles in the fields of social psychology and mental health policy. He recently coauthored a book on national trends in mental hospitalization.

Delores L. Parron, Ph.D., has been Associate Director for Special Populations, National Institute of Mental Health, since 1983. From 1978 to 1983 she was Associate Director of the Division of Mental Health and Behavioral Medicine, Institute of Medicine, National Academy of Sciences. She was a staff member of the President's Commission on Mental Health, 1977–1978, and Assistant Professor, Department of Psychiatry, Howard University College of Medicine, 1971–1978. She received her doctorate in Social Policy and Research from Catholic University of America. Her principal publications include *Health and Behavior, Frontiers of Research in the Biobehavioral Sciences* (1982), co-edited with David A. Hamburg and Glen R. Elliott; and *Mental Health Services in Primary Care Settings* (1980), with Frederic Solomon.

Richard Scheffler, Ph.D., is Professor of Health Economics and Public Policy in the Schools of Public Health and Public Policy, University of California, Berkeley, where he teaches health economics, health policy, and microeconomics. He is the Head of the Health Policy and Administration Program and the Director of the concurrent degree program in Health Policy in the Schools of Public Policy and Public Health. He also holds faculty appointments in the Department of Dental Public Health and Hygiene, School of Dentistry, University of California, San Francisco, and is an affiliated faculty member of the School of Business Administration at Berkeley and the Institute for Health Policy Studies, University of California, San Francisco. He is the Director of the Research Program in Health Economics in the Institute for Business and Economic Research, School of Business Administration, University of California, Berkeley.

Acknowledgments

We would like to acknowledge the assistance of Howard Rome for stimulating and urging us to put this volume together. He is a rare teacher, mentor, and friend. We would also like to thank Carl Eisdorfer for his friendship and encouragement. The book is dedicated to our teachers, Karl Menninger, Ed Greenwood, Bob Felix, and the late Gordon Derner.

LEONARD J. DUHL
NICHOLAS A. CUMMINGS

1

Introduction:
The Emergence of the
Mental Health Complex

Leonard J. Duhl
Nicholas A. Cummings
James J. Hynes

INTRODUCTION

This volume is addressed to all of the actors in the mental health
arena. Many of them, including psychiatrists, sense turmoil and
potential crisis. The crisis is real. The potential for a dramatic
shift to a new ballgame of mental health has never been greater.
We do not know who the power hitters will be, nor do we know
where the new ballpark will be. We only know that the game
will change.

In this lead-off chapter, we will examine some of the major
issues and tentatively suggest ways to deal with the stress
and change. Subsequent chapters will expand upon the issues
and provide a sense of direction for all of us in the mental
health field.

Complex, interrelated changes are occurring around us more

and more. As Capra (1) has noted, the extent of interrelatedness between fields has swelled to the point where changes in one field of endeavor are paralleled by changes in other fields. The health economist, Victor Fuchs (2), has also acknowledged the phenomenon and suggested, as Capra does in the title of his book, that we are at a turning point. According to Capra (3), at such a turning point the interdisciplinary qualities of our academic and professional pursuits will become self-evident. We must recognize, however, that massive and, at times, convulsive change has to occur before we reach such a turning point.

This volume arises out of concern with the massive changes many in the field of mental health have been experiencing. But instead of responding to such change with apprehension, distrust, and cynicism, this volume seeks to alert the professions to the parameters of the change it is experiencing and, in so doing, to suggest responses that will secure a better future for the provision of mental health services. We hope we will then be able to view the changes about us as ones leading to an optimistic future.

The mental health field, like other fields, is struggling to understand the sources of stress that are increasingly shaping its ability to meet the mental health needs of the population. Without such an understanding, the field will become more fragmented and the problem of poor services will be exacerbated.

As we know from our clinical work, a history often suggests intervention points. Thus, in the following sections, an outline of the recent history of mental health services from the end of World War II to the present will be presented. This search for intervention points can act as a mediator of the stress brought on by change, and, therefore, may have therapeutic value. Elliot and Eisdorfer (4) and others have noted that mediation strategies often are more important in the coping process than the particular substantive issues at hand. This chapter will delineate some of the current external and internal stressors in the field, as well as their roles in the emergence of the "mental health complex." The chapter will conclude with a brief discussion of power and control, and ways we can respond to the current stressors.

HISTORY

Before World War II, the problems of mental health were relatively simple. There were "snakepits" (5) as hospitals. The treatment of the mentally ill had not changed philosophically since the Middle Ages. "Treatment" was a means of social control wherein the deviant were shepherded off to large anonymous institutional warehouses. Indeed, these were total institutions (6) in the most pernicious sense. Changes and reforms came slowly. Whenever large-scale change did occur, the impetus for it came from outside the field.

A huge crisis, a world war, *had* to occur before any significant changes in mental health could occur. The optimism that symbolized the post–World War II era strongly influenced the future of many social programs, including mental health ones. The idea of planning, although already bolstered by the social and economic failures of the Depression, was part of this optimism and carried the idea that we, as a society, could control the future course of events. This applied as much to the returning military personnel as it did to the casualties of our society, the destitute. Thus the seeds for a more humanistic approach to social deviance were sown in the postwar era. We could no longer blame the victims (7). It is not surprising, then, that the 1946 founding legislation for the National Institute of Mental Health (NIMH) included not only provisions for rehabilitation of the mentally ill, but also, most importantly, provisions for the prevention of mental illness (8). In retrospect, this seems like a trivial statement; but it is important to recognize the historical context in which this legislation was drafted.

Despite the McCarthyism of the 1950s, postwar optimism carried over to facilitate the growth of the community mental health movement. The field began to differentiate, and more and more professionals joined the cause of mental health. One indicator of this growing interest is in the increased number of people on the membership list of the American Psychological Association. At the end of World War II there were only a few thousand, but by the late 1970s the numbers had increased to nearly a hundred thousand (9).

Of course, the rapid change in the mental health professions was encouraged by state legislatures and Congress, as well as by presidential commissions and private foundations (10). Vast increases in funding redefined the "game" of mental health concerns. The adoption of Medicare and Medicaid shifted financial control away from the National Institute of Mental Health. The Department of Health, Education and Welfare and third-party administrators assumed much more of the financial control. Administrators and economists began to exercise much more influence. At the same time, major developments in psychopharmacology changed patients, programs, hospitals, staffs, families, and communities. There was much optimism. In retrospect, we might say there was too much optimism.

By the 1960s, mental health was no longer a problem of "snakepits," nor was the problem owned by the psychiatrists of the large institutions. It became a social policy concern and involved a broad spectrum of newly arrived actors. And as more actors arrived, different professional languages developed. Communication became more difficult. Community participation requirements of many of the poverty and civil rights programs, although extremely important, added even more languages. The problem of communication intensified.

The events of the 1960s and early 1970s moved mental health away from the archaic linear model that had characterized it for so many years. As more and more professions became involved, it became apparent we were moving toward a complex inquiring system, in which no single profession could control the events in the field. Indeed, those external to the field (e.g., the economists) seemed to be influencing internal events more and more.

The notion of a complex of mental health stems from the ideas posited earlier on the growing interrelatedness of disciplines and economic sectors. The functional interrelatedness of economic sectors is not a new concept. The military-industrial complex (11) was defined in the late 1950s and early 1960s, while the medical-industrial complex (12) came to be defined by Relman in the late 1970s and early 1980s.

It was possible to define these complexes by reinterpreting the history and streams of influence of the respective fields. This possibility exists for mental health and speaks to the phenomenology surrounding the social construction of problems and reality (13). It is now possible to define a "mental health complex" in which there is less control, but greater interdependence among the array of fields in the complex. The complex will be more succinctly defined as we move toward a turning point.

Loss of control is one of the major reasons we have chosen to issue this volume. We must attempt to develop dialogue with our professional counterparts in hopes of dealing better with the task of providing improved care for the mentally disabled.

STRESS

The movement toward a mental health complex depends partially on the ways current stressors are mediated. For convenience and clarity, stressors are described as "internal" and "external."

Internally, the stressors come from three streams of thought: (1) biomedical, (2) psychological, and (3) psychosocial. Externally, the stressors come primarily from (1) economics, (2) politics, (3) demographics, and (4) the creation of self-help and de-professionalization movements.

Internal Stress Factors

Biomedical
Biomedical research continues to provide information and explanations for many mental health phenomena. From the dopamine etiological hypothesis on schizophrenia to gene markers for depression, the biomedical community is making important discoveries. Financial support for biomedical research will probably continue at present or greater levels in the future.

Within psychiatry, biomedical thinking is certainly on the rise. More and more of those going into psychiatry these days seem to do so more for biomedical than for psychotherapy concerns. Other indicators can be seen in the increase in brain chemistry research and the rise in psychoimmunology. For practicing psychiatrists, the emphasis on biology may mean that their future roles will be focused almost entirely on medication issues. As psychiatry medicalizes, psychotherapy will be left to the psychologists.

Psychological

The psychological stream of thought in mental health continues to develop new tributaries in the form of marriage, family, and child counseling (MFCC), expanded social-work roles, genetic counseling, and so forth. The development of these new roles is facilitated by the trend for less coverage of psychiatric services. For the third-party and out-of-pocket payers, lower-priced substitutes are more desirable.

Another factor behind the development of new professional roles is the growth of alternative health paradigms. The Esalen movement, humanistic psychology, and a variety of behaviorally oriented paradigms are questioning the assumptions and concepts behind other mental health paradigms. For some, values and practices are critically reexamined in light of such alternative explanations; and they experience stress.

Psychosocial

Another internal stressor on the field is the change occurring in the psychosocial field. As was noted above, there has been a burgeoning of specialty roles. They seem to recombine constantly with one another to form innovative perspectives. The focus on family systems (14), the workplace, ecological psychology (15), community networks (16), health psychology, and so on stimulates the development of new fields and mental health roles. These roles are necessary and inevitable in a changing world.

Psychosocial research and program planning competes with the biomedical community for financial support. Since a "curing" outlook is more likely to be supported politically, psychosocial agenda items are usually given less priority. Consequently, mental health professionals interested in psychological and environmental etiologies become threatened in their professional roles. Territoriality/turfism develops and fragments services and professionals. The more significant issues of ecological interdependence become clouded.

All around us there are increasing numbers of homeless people. Their presence is a direct reflection of our inability to care for the "walking" mentally ill (17). Although mental health moves toward a complex, a system, it is not doing very well with case management and issues of long-term care. Even though there are more professional roles and paradigms, we are just learning the need for appropriate mixing of needs and resources (both professional and self-help). Clearly, we must abandon some of our professional concerns if we are to explore new roles and participate in the evolving mental health complex.

The nature–nuture controversy may continue as an intellectual pursuit, but in so far as providing appropriate services to the population, the stance should be one of pragmatism.

External sources of change and stress have fueled the debate as well.

External Stress Factors

Economics

The economic *Zeitgeist* of today is determining the nature of mental health service delivery. Economic reasoning is increasingly being applied to questions about current and future mental health service levels, how they are to be delivered, and who will pay. Cost-containment arguments are powerful these days. They characterize much of the political climate, since much political power is built on cost-containment reasoning. Additionally, the advent of diagnosis-related groups (DRGs) and prepaid plans suggests movement toward capitated systems (18). Providers will have to relinquish some of their traditional decision-making responsibilities.

Politics

Of course, the politics of mental health includes many issues. The politics of mental health in California revolves around the issues of block granting from state to county and the subsequent controversies of cost shifting and patient dumping.

Block grants from state to counties are turning responsibility for mental health programs over to the Board of Supervisors. The decisions at this level, in all of the counties around the state, will increasingly influence the breadth and depth of state-supported mental health programs. Better accounting procedures and appropriate economies of scale may arise out of the state/county shift, but it is critically important to develop accounting systems that will indicate the flow of clients through the system and indicate the overall effects of our interventions on the population at need. At present, we have no way to track the usage patterns of either individuals or the larger population. The Legislative Analyst's Office can tell us nothing more than where the money in the system comes from, where it is spent, and the changes in the mental health budget from year to year (19). Whether there is a dumping phenomenon or cost shifting to the county, or even whether services are deteriorating, cannot be statistically demonstrated because there is no data. Unfortunately, from the state's point of view, if there is no data, there is no problem. Most of us in the field, however, do not need data to claim worsening services. It is happening all around, and we seem to hear more and more horror stories on poor services (20), substandard living conditions, and homelessness (21).

The political input on mental health issues in California is beginning to be based on a law-and-order mentality. The governor's 1984–85 budget proposal included hefty increases in appropriations for mental hospitals, while community-based programs continue to experience decreases in budget appropriations. The concept of aftercare services and planning is not a high political priority. This indicates something of a shift in basic social and political values. While only some of us may experience the stress of de-professionalization, all of us will be increasingly besieged with the question of who will do therapy.

Demographics

We are an aging population. As the "rectangularization of the life expectancy curve" continues, there will be more chronic mental disorders. This may mean totally different types of services than those presently available. The emphasis may change to long-term care rather than "cure" as it becomes evident that many of the needs of the elderly are mental health needs.

In California, projections (22) suggest a future population dominated by two distinct groups, the elderly white population and the young Chicano population. Services will surely have to change to meet the needs of these emerging populations. The tensions bound to develop between these groups over issues of who pays for what may require new types of mental health services. Professional roles will differentiate markedly in this scenario.

Self-help and De-Professionalization

Paralleling the development of specialty roles in the last quarter of a century, there has been a backlash on the part of many mental health consumers. Most have experienced the revolving door of the institution and have come to the realization that they can take care of themselves. The use of community support networks and self-help (23) groups is increasing. The emphasis is more on management of disorders rather than cure. The self-help movement is necessary and will profoundly affect all of our professional roles.

The three internal stressors and the four external stressors listed above should be considered by all mental health professionals. They will guide the emergence of our future roles.

RESPONDING TO STRESS

The intensity of the stressors on professional roles seems to be associated with each profession's overall ability to control events in its field. Seeley (24) has noted that mental health connotes the extent of one's ability to control surrounding events. Perhaps this connotation applies as much to the mental health complex. The greater the control, the less the stress and consequent sense of crisis; while less control means greater stress and sense of crisis. Observations seem to lend some credence to this notion.

Psychiatrists, relatively powerful and controlling in the mental health complex, are less moved in their roles as stressors mount, while, in sharp contrast, other professionals, such as MFCCs, genetic counselors, social workers, and health psychologists are much more affected by the stressors. Some professionals will have to scramble quickly in order to survive in the emerging environment. As new roles emerge, we should try to avoid the winners–losers way of thinking. This is not the desirable process. We must think ecologically, adaptively, and cooperatively. Win-win (25) situations are conceivable in ecological systems. As a complex, our health is then redefined as arising out of a social context in which there is harmonious interaction of the systems (26) of mental health. Thus, the professionals in the mental health complex must begin to find self-interest in each other.

The seven stressors delineated above are highly interconnected and affect one another. Capra (27) sees this type of interrelatedness as contributing to the development of "para" societies. As we move toward a "para" society, seemingly disparate areas become increasingly intertwined. We will be forced to examine fundamental questions, such as "What is health?" and "What is education?" Such inquiry speaks to the complex, interdisciplinary overlap among all areas of knowledge. The implications on the sociology of knowledge are enormous. Our sense of finiteness and holism expands.

The changes and issues we speak of in this volume prompt both crisis and opportunity. The better we understand the stressors, the more we can participate in the emerging world. This chapter does not contend that internal or external stressors are necessarily bad. Responses to the stress may be either adaptive or maladaptive. For example, economics allows for the introduction of cost efficiency and competition leading to, perhaps, doing more with less. It also allows for the creation of competitive local programs, which may be either public or private. New forms of organization and management are possible and may successfully challenge our old concepts of services planning by leading us to paths previously uncontemplated. Poignant examples of such are the Health Maintenance Organizations (HMOs), such as Rockridge in the San Francisco Bay area or Montefiore in the Bronx. Other novel forms of institutional organizations, such as On Lok, a social HMO in San Francisco, are being created in many other places. Each has service characteristics and the respective professional staffing and client characteristics determined more by locally defined variables than by removed centralized administrative units.

These organizations, which have responded to stress successfully, share several characteristics:

1. They are non-guild oriented. Responsibilities are delegated according to a collegial model based on "redundancy" characteristics (28). For example, a case is assigned to staff not so much on the basis of professional roles, but on who can best meet the needs of the particular client. Collegial models facilitate a continuous process of mixing and matching needs and resources. In the long run, they are more cost-effective. Can the professions of the mental health complex afford to find solutions on their own? The evidence is to the contrary.

2. They are systems oriented in their thinking and look to mental health needs as existing in a larger context. Mental health then becomes defined as meaning homes and jobs and

friends. Do we go the route of separating out medical, psycho-logical, and social aspects from each other, or do we go the route of comprehensive programs?

3. They take on greater amounts of financial risk. This allows more local decision making about mental health resources. According to Richard Zawadski (29) of On Lok in San Francisco, "the price of freedom is financial risk." As providers start sharing ownership responsibilities in the organizations they work in, there may be a conflict of interest. That is, will decision making be based on patients or profits?

4. They attempt to reconceptualize the problems they deal with as much more than professional conceptualizations. Perhaps they realize that "If the only tool you have is a hammer, then all your problems are nails" (30).

These are just a few of the characteristics that are readily perceivable. They represent some of the ways organizations have responded successfully to the stressors around them. All the actors in the mental health complex should take heed of these characteristics, and look for ways they can learn from them.

We have spent much time concerned with issues of research, politics, and systems. The clients, their families, and their communities are hardly mentioned. Their self-defined needs are the most important inputs. Some of these needs were eloquently expressed by Howard Harp, of the California Network of Mental Health Clients. They involve housing, jobs, empowerment, and less drugs. When these needs are met, there are greater possibilities for independent living. The key to getting these needs met, as expressed by Mr. Harp, is empowerment:

> . . . powerlessness further reinforces dependent behavior and poor self-image, which is ultimately hazardous to the client's mental health. The power to control one's own life, which can also be defined as freedom, is very positive and self-affirming—good for one's mental health. Programs that encourage independence are few and far between. Mental health related programs and residences should be encouraged to involve present and former clients in their operation and decision making structure on a day to day basis. Clients and residents should have more opportunities to make decisions about their programs. Many of us, like myself, spent years in places where all the decisions were made for us. The

ability to make decisions is vital to being independent. You cannot learn how to do it until you start doing it (31).

The following chapters will touch upon some of the points we have made here. Taken together, they represent a call for action.

REFERENCES

1. Capra, F. (1982). *The turning point*. New York: Simon and Schuster.
2. Fuchs, V. (1974). *Who shall live?: Health, economics and social choice*. New York: Basic Books.
3. Capra, F. (1982). *The turning point*. New York: Simon and Schuster.
4. Elliot, G. R., & Eisdorfer, C. (Eds.). (1982). *Stress and human health: Analysis and implications for research*. New York: Springer Publishing Co.
5. Deutsch, A. (1949). *The mentally ill in America*. New York: Columbia University Press.
6. Goffman, E. (1961). *Asylums*. New York: Doubleday and Co.
7. Ryan, W. (1976). *Blaming the victim*. New York: Vintage Books.
8. The 1946 National Mental Health Act.
9. Krasner, L. (1979, March). Lecture given at S.U.N.Y. at Stony Brook, NY.
10. Joint Commission for Mental Health. (1961). *Actions for mental health*, Washington, DC: Government Printing Office.
11. Eisenhower, D. (1960, January). *Presidential farewell address*.
12. Relman, A. (1980). The new medical-industrial complex. *New England Journal of Medicine, 303*(17), 996–998.
13. Schon, D. (1983). *The reflective practitioner: How professionals think in action*. New York: Basic Books.
14. Rueveni, U., Speck, R., & Speck, J. (Eds.). (1982). *Therapeutic intervention: Healing strategies for human systems*. New York: Human Services Press.
15. Fairweather, G. (1972). *Social change: The challenge to survival*. Morristown, NJ: General Learning Press.
16. Pilisuk, M. (1982). Delivery of social support: The social inoculation. *American Journal of Orthopsychiatry, 52*, 20–30.
17. Talbot, J. (1984, May) *Response to the president's address*. Paper presented at the 137th annual meeting of the American Psychiatric Association, San Diego, CA.
18. Ginzberg, E. (1984). *The monetarization of medical care. New England Journal of Medicine, 310*(18), 1162–1165.
19. Legislative Analyst's Office of the State of California. *Report to the select committee on mental health*. Sacramento, CA.
20. Davenport, M. (1984, April). *Testimony before the select committee on mental health*. Sacramento, CA.

21. Farr, R. (1984, May). *Testimony before the California state legislature's select committee on mental health.* San Diego, CA.
22. Hayes-Bautista, D., Schinck, W., & Chapa, J. (1984). *California's demographic future: Issues for planners. Westplan,* Issue #7.
23. Katz, A., Levin, L., & Holst, E. (1976). *Self-care: Lay initiatives in health.* New York: Prodist.
24. Seeley, J. (1967). *The Americanization of the unconscious.* New York: International Science Press.
25. Fisher, R., & Ury, W. (1981). *Getting to yes: Negotiating agreement without giving in.* Boston: Houghton-Mifflin.
26. Blum, H. (1981). *Planning for health: Generics for the eighties.* New York: Human Sciences Press.
27. Capra, F. (1982). *The turning point.* New York: Simon and Schuster.
28. Landau, M. (1973). On the concept of a self-correcting organization. *Public Administration Review,* Issue #6.
29. Interview with Zawadski at On Lok, San Francisco, CA, April, 1984.
30. Maslow, A. Personal communication.
31. Harp, H. (1984, April). *Testimony before the select committee on mental health.* San Diego, CA.

2

The Social Context of Change

Robert A. Aldrich

INTRODUCTION

The purpose of this chapter is to consider the nature and meaning of the social changes that have been occurring in the United States in recent years. This is necessary because the character of a society enormously influences the mental well-being of its citizens. Population dynamics (demography) will be emphasized, because of the basic role it plays in determining values, along with economics. There also are worldwide demographic shifts over which we in the United States have little control. These, too, are having an impact on our values, economy, and mental attitudes. We are nearly all economy watchers, but few of us watch demography. The record suggests that more realism and better forecasting of the effects of social change would come from closer attention to population dynamics.

What I am expressing here is the idea that the epidemiology of mental well-being very likely is linked closely to social structure and function. Thus the ability to adapt to change in society may aid mental well-being, while inability to adapt may often be manifested in mental illness. The adaptability of human beings to a culture different from their own varies with individuals, age, and sex. Many of us have experienced cultural shock while traveling in foreign nations, or even in unfamiliar parts of the United States.

An experience with cultural shock is temporary, although the event remains notably long in one's memory. One's adaptability was exceeded, causing anxiety and discomfort. Humankind is not infinitely adaptable, as we have come to realize; nor can high technology compensate for limitations to adaptation in a great many instances, although good progress has been achieved for the physically handicapped by advances in medicine, biology, and engineering. As change continues we are compelled to abandon previously successful ways of doing things in favor of better methods for accommodating to rapid change. The prime question is: What are these changes and how can human beings accommodate to them? Critical observations of social change and population dynamics may provide us with the clues we need for advancing mental well-being and reducing those factors in society that are the most difficult for people to adjust to.

WORLD POPULATION

It is estimated that the world population is approximately 4.76 billion and that by the year 2000 there will be a population of 6.25 billion (1). Estimates of this kind differ in minor ways, as one might expect, but there is good general agreement on the size and structure of world population. Some specific examples follow to illustrate the dramatic force of population shifts. Additional data can be obtained from the World Bank Reports (2). In addition, the 1982 census of the People's Republic of China has just been made available through the National Academy of Sciences in Washington, D.C.

- Mexico City is projected to become the world's largest city, with a population of 32 million by the end of the century.
- China presently has a population of 650,000 million who are under the age of thirty.

- Average rates of world population growth have been slow-ing, with developing countries dropping from a rate of 2.4% in 1960 to 2.0% in 1984 (3).
- Most of the Western world has reached population replace-ment levels or is approaching it.
- At the end of the century, the world population will be 6.25 billion, an increment of almost 1.5 billion.
- If the current policies in China for one child per family are successful, China will still account for 1.2 billion of the 6.25 billion at century's end.
- The United Nations estimated in 1980 that the U.S. popula-tion would grow to about 270 million, from 234 million, by the year 2000.
- The UN also predicts that world population will reach "no growth" by approximately the year 2095, when world pop-ulation will have reached just over 10 billion and births equal deaths.
- The U.S. death rate is now higher than China's. China has a much younger population.

INFLUENCES ON HUMAN VALUES

In effect, the world is experiencing a massive population change, placing heavy burdens upon the less developed countries, whose resources are far too limited for the needs of their citizens. This fact poses questions of a strategic nature for the well-developed countries who occupy the same planet. Nations such as the United States, Japan, and those of Western Europe and Scandi-navia all have low birth rates accompanied by rapidly aging populations; they consume a much larger percent of the world's resources in proportion to their population than do the less developed countries. The latter are expressing strong arguments for shifting more of these resources in their direction.

The impacts of world population changes on human values have been explored by Dr. Jonas Salk (4, 5, 6). He draws an analogy between the growth curve of microorganisms in a closed system and the population growth of human beings. The familiar sigmoid growth curve (Figure 2.1) for microorganisms, after an initial rapid growth, slows and bends to the right when

Figure 2.1 The sigmoid growth curve for
microorganisms in a closed system.

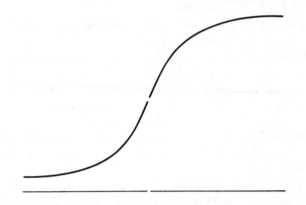

essential nutrients are in short supply and become limiting
factors. He proposes that the population growth curve for human beings might follow the same principles (4), as it seems to
be doing. This idea implies that limiting growth factors on a
world basis—such as food, energy, clean water—may force
changes in human values in order for humankind to survive.

Table 2.1 lists, under column *A*, several human values that
have had at least two generations of major influence in the
United States, while column *B* represents the direction in which
these values may be shifting. It is of some interest that when this
table was presented recently to a Japanese group of professional
and business leaders, one of them commented that the values
under column *B* are held by Japanese and, in his opinion, are at

Table 2.1 Changing Values

A	B
Competition	Cooperation
Parts	Whole
Absolute	Balance
Power	Consensus
Independence	Interdependence
Individual	Group

least partly responsible for the ability of certain Japanese industries to excel over those in the United States. My point is that population dynamics can have an effect on the values of a society and this, in turn, can influence industrial performance, economics, and survival. It is well to remember that Japan reduced its birthrate by nearly 50 percent in the immediate post–World War II years, an achievement necessary for national survival.

THE UNITED STATES

Population Changes

The list of important population changes in the United States is long. Those that appear to have considerable potential for effecting changes in mental well-being include:

1. The population is rapidly aging, as shown in Figure 2.2. The low numbers of children at the base of the demographic map (left side) must be compared to the large base of a developing country (right side). Projections into the first two decades of the next century suggest there will be shortages of young adults for the work force, which will probably cause restrictions on those wishing to retire at age sixty-five. Older men and women may need to be retained in the work force. It is also likely that financing their retirement will no longer be possible under the same conditions provided today.

2. Family structure is diversifying through divorce, cohabitation, and a variety of other family configurations that include both adults and children. These innovations will affect child and youth behavior in as yet unpredictable ways. Traditional concepts of family security and support systems are being modified rapidly.

3. Women have entered the work force in large numbers. About 50 percent of women with children are working. This profound social change brings two incomes into many homes, while placing limits on the amount of time and effort that can be devoted to child rearing and other home-related activities. Working women who are single are faced with a level of responsibility that can be crushing—to earn a living, keep up a

Figure 2.2 Demographic chart of developed versus developing countries. Population distribution by age and sex, 1975 (medium variant).

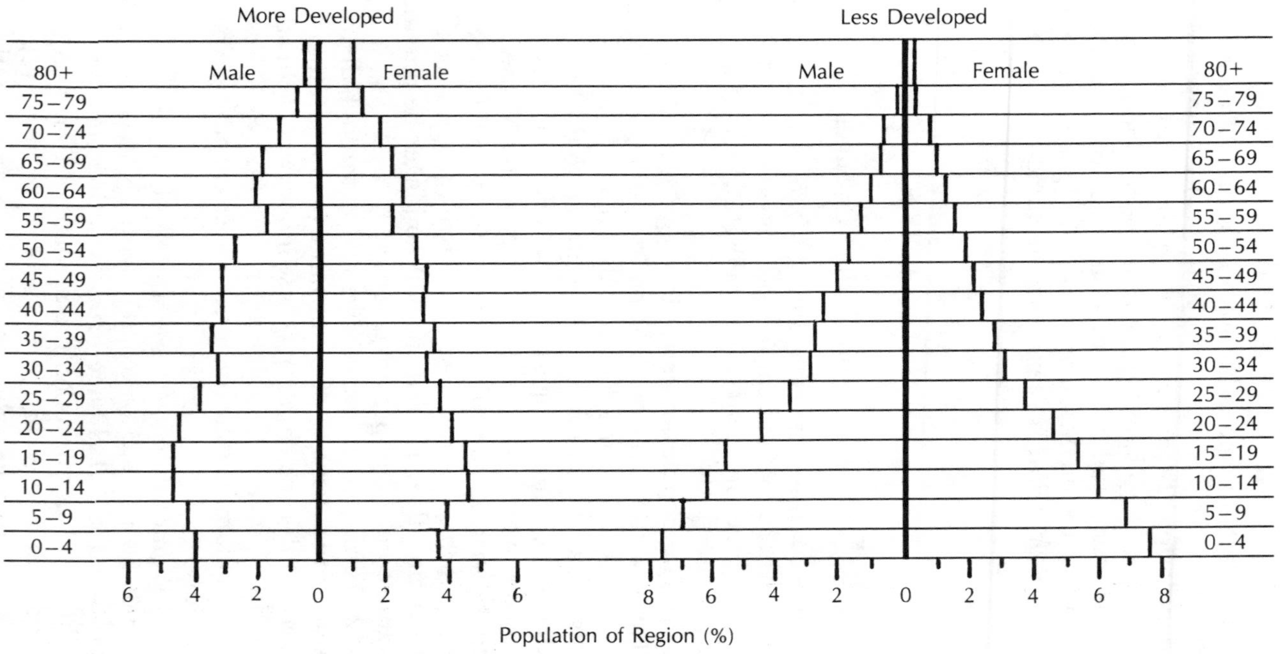

home, raise a child, and have some time for personal life is more than a full-time task, leading many into economic poverty.

4. The population is shifting toward the Southwest. In 1983, the Census Bureau reported that Chicago has been replaced by Los Angeles as the second-largest city in the United States. The Southwest is the recipient of very large numbers of people migrating from Mexico and Asian countries. Articles from European newspapers and a British magazine, *The Economist,* express apprehension over the growing interest by the United States in the Pacific Rim region and the huge markets located there. Thoughtful men and women are asking whether this will reduce American interest in Europe, with all the attendant political and economic implications. The traditional special relationships between Europe and the United States that are so deeply rooted are being threatened.

5. Urbanization is perhaps the single most characteristic phenomenon of the United States in this century. Although our agricultural productivity is the wonder of the world, we are no longer a rural nation. The great majority of Americans have moved to work and live in urban settings.

Virtually all of our cities are also industrialized, contrasting with nonindustrialized cities in less developed nations. We are well equipped with new and high technology that constantly flows from many years of scientific development, while less developed nations lag far behind in technology, scientific development, and economic resources.

Communications

Electronic connections between us bring information about happenings anywhere in the world, within a few minutes of the event, to citizens of every age. Everyday communication with family and friends, business or professional men and women, is easily available and inexpensive. We are like a single large community, linked as we are by telecommunications that improve the efficiency of our homes, offices, manufacturing, and government, provide greater safety and security, and create new forms of business activity such as computers and related services.

Nuclear Weaponry and Industry

Nuclear weaponry and industry are two completely new, man-made sources of energy.

Nuclear weaponry has the power to destroy entire cities and nations, as well as the potential for ending life as we know it on this planet. Weaponry is now an investment of such size for the major powers that it successfully competes for national funds needed elsewhere for human services, capital investment, new industries, maintenance of the infrastructure (water, sewage, roads, etc), scientific development, and education. Nuclear weaponry and industry have both become politicized in the United States, distracting thousands of able individuals from their normal activities. But the greatest impact of nuclear weaponry is the fear and anxiety in the minds of children, youth, and adults. Fear about the future and a feeling of impending disaster are shared by many who believe they have lost control of their lives.

Nuclear industrial plants generating electric power could be a resource for less developed as well as developed nations. However, neither safe disposal of nuclear waste nor reasonable building and operating costs exist at present.

Health and Health Care

Americans perceive health as a more complex concept than medicine. They see medicine as an important part of health and health care, but the two terms are not synonymous. Health is a right in the minds of most Americans. People expect that the professions and facilities that make up health care will be organized, managed, and accessible to them at a cost they can afford. Public pressure is now forcing both the government and the private sectors who own and manage health care to invent new ways of preventing illness, promoting and maintaining health, and intervening to treat disease.

Knowledge about health is booming. Browsing in a bookstore quickly settles any doubts about the general public's interest in health. There are hundreds of books on wellness, diet, exercise, fitness, the disease of the month, air and water, pollution, as well as do-it-yourself guides to self-care. As the population ages, books about the infirmities that can occur in later life are blossoming. And importantly, many of these are focused on the social aspects of living in one's older years. We seem to be entering an era when long life is the norm and quality of that life throughout its span is the goal. Health as a continuing process over the life span and thus a part of human development is a relatively new idea (7).

Crime and Antisocial Behavior

Crime and antisocial behavior have been a part of human society for thousands of years. It may be, as some have proposed, that this is a characteristic of *Homo sapiens* requiring constant efforts by society to control. Whatever the merit of this point of view, the fact remains that crimes against individuals and social institutions in the United States continue to increase. In spite of vigorous efforts at law enforcement, our prisons and jails are overcrowded, criminal courts are falling behind in their work load, and citizens believe they are at risk on the streets and in their homes.

Each evening the television news leads off with a body count of murders, assaults (mugging, rape), burglaries, arson, riots, vandalism, violent accidents (automobiles, trains), and sometimes an earthquake or flood if nature cooperates. We are made aware of the frailties of leading citizens and elected officials in fine detail, with rarely a word or scene depicting those who make up most of the tapestry of society by their reliable, constructive daily efforts.

Recent visitors from Scandinavia recounted the average Nordic's view of the United States gained through the media, including motion pictures: streets swarming with armed police who shoot without warning anyone in their way, widespread abuse of drugs among children and youth, rampant corruption in business and government circles, and very little safety in one's own home. We appear to project to ourselves and to others a pattern of antisocial behavior. There is undoubtedly some truth behind all of this, but is it realistic or even ethical to expose one aspect of our society without the others that counterbalance it? This phenomenon is part of social change, and a very long way from the picture we had of ourselves and our country earlier in the century. The days of unlocked doors at home, neighborly cooperation, courtesy, civility, and openness to new acquaintances are disappearing.

Terrorism is another form of crime and antisocial behavior. The United States has been relatively free of this activity, except for a wave of air piracy (hijacking). But other parts of the world are suffering from bombings and assassinations, engendering predictions that we will soon have to cope with terrorists. One encouraging note was the way the Olympic Games were conducted safely in Los Angeles, where security arrangements were extraordinarily effective. It remains to be seen whether our present society can prevent or contain terrorism.

Environmental Pollution

Pollution today has taken a different form from that of fifty years ago. Highly toxic new synthetic chemicals, radioactivity, excessive noise, and even electronic beams are being targeted for control because of their potential damage to human beings. The burning of fossil fuels is now on a scale that many believe is damaging lakes, rivers, and forests through fallout of acid rain. Some of these forms of pollution travel long distances into countries abutting the polluting sources. Canada is pointing to industrial plants and power-generating stations in the mid-western United States as the sources of acid rain in eastern Canada. Environmental pollution has become a global problem, as experienced air travelers have known for several decades. The layer of polluted air a few thousand feet above the ground has become much more dense and extensive.

Toxic chemicals have already forced residential communities to relocate because of the discovery that their housing developments were constructed on landfill containing dangerous toxic materials. These experiences have led to federal legislation and appropriations intended to clean up known sites. Greater control is being sought by municipalities and states in order to prevent land contamination by waste disposal. Lakes, rivers, salt water bays, and harbors are being studied for pollution. The fishing industry has just discovered that environmental pollution can affect supplies of anadromous fish (e.g., salmon) by poisoning their spawning habitat. The forest industry has been severely criticized for its aerial spraying of pesticides. This practice has been limited as to both the chemicals permitted, which must not be harmful to human beings or animals, and the areas that can be sprayed. During the war in Vietnam the defoliant Agent Orange was sprayed from aircraft on soldiers operating in the field. It is claimed to be responsible for some defective offspring of these men. Litigation over these claims is in the courts, but a few veterans have already received government payments.

Urban Children and Youth

The majority of children and youth are growing up today in an urban environment. The needs of this age range have not been systematically designed in America's large cities. Some add-ons or adjustments have been made, but the fact remains that our major cities are designed by and for adults. Rarely are the wishes of children and youth considered, and practically never are their opinions asked. This is far different from the family farm or the small rural community, whose daily affairs are visible to a child and comprehensible as a model of how human beings interact in a variety of situations. The child reared in a small rural place has an image of a community as a whole, while the city-reared child can never master more than a few fragments of these huge communities.

I believe that urban-raised children and youth are at a disadvantage in this regard and that the difficulties urban children are having may be in part the result. It may be much easier for the rural child or youth to expand his or her concept of the community as a whole into a much larger community, the big city, than for the urban child who has never grasped the concept of community. And for this reason, we should start educating our urban children and their families in a different way. They need to learn urban skills (traffic, safety on the street, shopping techniques, neighborliness, city geography, bus transport, etc.), what their parents do at work, and where that work is located. We must begin to ask children what they wish the city provided them and be prepared to listen and to act on their ideas. Cities that initiate programs of participation by children and youth in planning will learn that young people take inquiries seriously and offer sensible ideas. Their part in planning is absolutely essential if we are to build in them a feeling of identity for "their" city. It should be a part of their growth and development. My expectation is that where this process is encouraged, the involved young men and women will later become important sources of civic leadership when they have assumed responsible adult roles in society. They will be the future cadre of citizens who care about the city, serving as an example for following generations.

An experiment along these lines is going on in Seattle, Washington. It is called "KidsPlace," a term suggested and chosen by Seattle kids. The project conducted research about the city as seen through the eyes of children and youth and presented their findings and ideas at a national conference in April 1985. The purpose of the conference was to establish an agenda for the city. Thirty-one issues are being addressed, such as schools, housing, transportation, and waterfront development. More than a score of good ideas have emerged already, and there will be more. At least one of these suggestions has been carried out by city government. A carefully constructed survey of all school-children, attending both independent and public schools, is complete. The results in terms of participation leave no doubt about the survey's being taken seriously. Good sense and ideas most adults would not have thought about characterize the responses. There is a "Hawthorne Effect" happening. Just the fact that something on this scale with this focus is going on appears to induce businesses, volunteer organizations, professionals, foundations, and government to join in some aspect of the project or examine their own activity from the standpoint of how it might be seen by children or youths. It can be a start toward bringing more congruence into the relationship of our young and our cities, with benefits to all.

IN TRANSITION

What does all of this change mean? Where will it lead? How will it influence mental well-being? Is there a process that helps to predict social change? These are a few of the questions needing answers. It is not so much a new ballgame that we are engaged in, but a new ballpark, different players, new rules—and not a game at all!

We are all in transition, and so are our politics, societies, cultures, and institutions. There is no previous model known for what is happening today. We have no source of prior experience to guide us in the immediate future. So, in this sense, we have become both the research director and the guinea pig on this earth. The challenges facing us are so complex that they may feature millions of variables requiring the use of statistical technologies, probability theory, genetic laws, and theories of atomic motion. "Disorganized complexity" is the term used by Warren Weaver for challenges of this nature (8).

The new ballpark is the world, the different players are the world population, and the new rules are changed value systems. And most compelling of all is the fact that we are now playing for keeps, with human survival and evolution as the winning score.

How long we will be in transition is impossible to estimate when every year new archeological–anthropological discoveries move our origins further back in time. The positive side of humankind's story is continuing evolution. I believe we have among us some examples of further evolved human beings. They are extraordinary men and women who seem to have capabilities considerably beyond others. Perhaps we should follow the principle that all should advance evolutionary development. This may be the ethical direction to take.

Finally, we can put to good use the knowledge that we now have about human life-span development. People need to learn more about themselves, beginning in elementary school and continuing throughout all stages of life. Figure 2.3 is a model

Figure 2.3 A schematic portrayal of human life-span development.

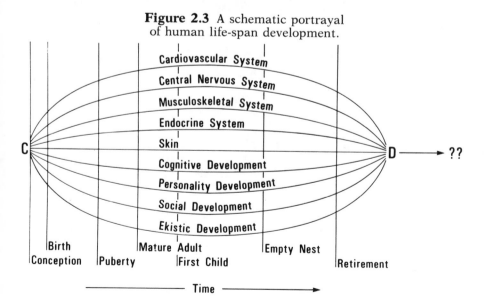

Cardiovascular System
Central Nervous System
Musculoskeletal System
Endocrine System
Skin
Cognitive Development
Personality Development
Social Development
Ekistic Development

C   D ⟶ ??

Birth   Mature Adult   Empty Nest
Conception   Puberty   First Child   Retirement

⟵ Time ⟶

constructed for college and graduate students that has proved to be easily understood in several cultures. Its use is described in detail in other publications (7, 9). Mental well-being may be the product of successful life-span human development.

REFERENCES

1. Population Reference Bureau, Inc., (1984). *1984 world population data sheet*. Washington, DC: Author.
2. The World Bank. (1984). *World development report 1984*. New York: Oxford University Press.
3. *The Economist*, July 14, 1984, p. 76–77.
4. Salk, J. E. (1973). *The survival of the wisest*. New York: Harper & Row, p. 124.
5. Salk, J. E., & Salk, J. *World population and human values—A new reality*. (1981). New York: Harper & Row, p. 170.
6. Salk, J. E. (1983). *Anatomy of reality—Merging of intuition and reason*. New York: Columbia University Press, p. 127.
7. Aldrich, R. A. (1977). Human life-span development, a life science for epoch B. In H. O. Hess (Ed.), *The nature of a humane society*, edited by H. Ober Hess, (pp. 171–185). Philadelphia: Fortress Press.
8. Weaver, W. (1948). Science and complexity. *The American Scientist*, 6, 536–544.
9. Moore, L. G., Van Arsdale, P., Glittenberg, J., & Aldrich, R. A. (1980). *The biocultural basis of health*. St. Louis: C. V. Mosby, p. 278.

3

The Federal
Mental Health Agenda

Shervert H. Frazier
Delores L. Parron

INTRODUCTION

Just as case histories are crucial to us in understanding how our patients have arrived at the crisis state in which we encounter them, events occurring both within and around the National Institute of Mental Health (NIMH) over its nearly forty years of existence are vital to understanding its current role in the mental health field and delineating its role in the "new ballgame" of mental health. Although Duhl, Cummings, and Hynes have pointed out, in Chapter 1, several significant benchmarks for the mental health field, the history of NIMH is important to appreciating the current federal mental health agenda.

NIMH HISTORY

The legislation authorizing the NIMH was signed by President Truman in 1946 in response to several impetuses: concern over the large number of men rejected for military duty in World War II as a result of mental disability; concern over professional staff shortages and deteriorating conditions in many public mental hospitals; and optimism over the potentials of science for solving a whole raft of medical, behavioral, social, and other problems.

Public Law 79-487 charged the National Institute of Mental Health to support and conduct research on the nature, treatment, and prevention of mental illness; to train mental health personnel; and to help states develop community-based mental health services. Given its service responsibilities, the NIMH could have been placed in the Bureau of State Services, but Congress determined that the treatment of mental illness would be furthered most effectively by an emphasis on research and research training, and the NIMH was placed in the National Institutes of Health.

For the following twenty or so years, the three legs—research, training, and services—kept pretty well in stride. Interest in community-based services continued to increase, boosted by both the advent of psychotropic medications and the increasing availability of highly trained professionals. In 1959, the Joint Commission on Mental Illness and Health recommended continued expansion of each of the areas. In the early 1960s, President Kennedy, in response to the findings of the Joint Commission, as well as to the urgings of a coterie of public health–oriented advisers, pushed successfully for the Federal Community Mental Health Centers Initiative.

Kennedy was also convinced of the need for research and aimed for a doubling of what was then being invested. The NIMH research budget grew rapidly in the late 1950s, in large part a reflection of congressional interest in advancing the emerging and promising field of psychopharmacology. From $8 million in 1956, it grew to $54 million in 1962 and to more than $90 million in 1965. Then two critical developments occurred.

One was passage of the Community Mental Health Centers (CMHC) legislation—construction grants in 1963, and staffing grants, under President Johnson, in 1965. A second was Johnson's pledge to apply scientific research to such social ailments as poverty, crime, urban problems, drug addiction, and alcoholism. A number of "Centers" were established within NIMH to coordinate research, special training initiatives, and service demonstration programs focused on these various problem areas.

These developments had various immediate and long-term effects. Immediately, large outlays for community mental health centers reduced the proportion of research as part of the total NIMH budget and, thus, its preeminence. In 1965, the research allocation was $91.5 million, and the services total was $10.6 million. Two years later, research had increased to $103.8 million, but services had surged to more than $94 million. This radical shift in the character of the Institute played a large part in prompting removal of NIMH from the exclusively research-oriented National Institutes of Health. After a few temporary placements in various health service bureaucracies, the Institute served as the rib from which the Alcohol, Drug Abuse, and Mental Health Administration (ADAMHA) was created in 1973.

Another effect of the mid-1960s policy decisions was to foster a perception some ten years later that the mental health research portfolio had become too diffuse. This view was held by people both within and outside the Institute who were concerned that the NIMH was placing inappropriate emphasis on topics that were only tenuously related to mental illness and mental health.

Yet another development crucial to the Institute's current position involved clinical training in the core mental health disciplines (psychiatry, psychology, social work, and nursing), which reached its peak in terms of dollars in 1969. The following year, the Nixon administration began to reassess the federal role in all health manpower education; with the involvement of Congress, this reassessment process was prolonged, and, in fact, continues to this day. NIMH currently maintains a modest budget in clinical training support—about $20 million per year—and the Institute interacts extensively and intensively with the field. This is important symbolically as well as substantively, insofar as NIMH contributes to curriculum development and other activities aimed at maintaining an adequate supply of mental health professionals with the capability of providing services to the mentally ill. Most recently, NIMH has shifted the emphasis of awards in support of clinical training toward preparation of professionals to serve children, adolescents, the elderly, and minority groups, rather than a simple discipline-focused distribution of funds as in the past. In line with the increasing state responsibilities in the delivery of mental health services, the Institute has directed funds toward state manpower development activities.

Block Grants for Alcohol, Drug Abuse, and Mental Health Services

With respect to an NIMH role in mental health services, the oft-amended but essentially continuous CMHC program was the subject of close scrutiny by President Carter's Commission on Mental Health in 1978. The outcome was enactment in 1980 of the Mental Health Systems Act, an extensive reformulation of the law that placed heavy emphasis on the needs of the chronically mentally ill. That act was, in effect, repealed with enactment of the Omnibus Budget Reconciliation Act of 1981.

Reorganization of the NIMH

Most recently, the rate of advance in the neurosciences and related disciplines, along with the increasingly precise understanding of the nature of distinct mental disorders, has motivated the NIMH to undertake a major reorganization in an effort to streamline its operations and thus provide greater organizational visibility for the Institute's support of basic brain and behavioral sciences research. Modifications of NIMH organizational structure in the past have enabled the Institute to continue to function at a high level of productivity and excellence, but they have also resulted in some duplication of effort and a blurring of the authority and responsibilities of many programs. The reorganization eliminates fragmentation and overlap by combining what are now separate research and research training organizations and focusing their efforts on today's important scientific fields (e.g., neurosciences, behavioral science, psychobiology); disorder/problem areas (e.g., schizophrenia, affective disorders, childhood and adolescent disorders, aging, and violence); and crosscutting concerns (e.g., epidemiology, treatment assessment, prevention, and minority group mental health concerns, including the development of minority scientists for careers in mental health research). This important shift in focus will enhance the Institute's efforts in areas of high priority.

Managing and Nurturing Research: Issues of Balance

Research is emerging as the Institute's major mission, and that research is increasingly biomedical. Contrary to some concerns, this trend is more the product of developments emanating from within the mental health field, particulary psychiatry, than from influences external to it.

Within the field, the shift began more than a decade ago. Perceptions that mental health research had become overly diffuse coincided with advances in a variety of areas that appeared to open "windows of opportunity" for research on mental illnesses. These included such areas as classification and diagnosis; the introduction of psychopharmacologic drugs; the twin and adoptive studies that served to verify a genetic element in major psychiatric disorders; advances in treatment, particularly of the affective disorders; new behavioral approaches to managing disorders; and others. But the window flung open the widest has been in the neurosciences. They are exciting, productive, and technologically based. They promise fundamental gains in our understanding of the substrates of illness and behavior. In certain areas, such as molecular biology, they have begun to narrow the gap between traditional notions of basic versus applied or clinical research.

By supporting the development of careers in mental health research and service delivery, NIMH has been able to create a cadre of skilled basic and clinical investigators in a wide range of biological, psychological, and social sciences who are eager to pursue opportunities to unravel the complexities of the burden of illness posed by mental disorders and to identify promising leads for promotion of mental health. As knowledge about and treatments for these disorders have improved, demands for new types of specially trained researchers have been created. For example, the provision of appropriate care delivered in the most efficient way possible requires skills in planning service systems, applying the principles of economics to the mental health sector, and identifying high-risk populations. Toward this end, the NIMH has encouraged the development of such highly specialized areas as mental health economics, mental health systems planning, program evaluation, and mental health epidemiology and statistics.

Recent research has demonstrated the importance of addressing transcultural issues in diagnosis and treatment (1, 2, 3). Demographic trends also indicate significant growth of the numbers of racial/ethnic minorities in the population. These trends signal the need to pay attention to the variables of race and ethnicity in research on mental disorders and the design of a responsive mental health system. Researchers who are members of minority groups are needed to provide important perceptions of what it is to be a member of a minority group. These perceptions, even in the biomedical sciences, can be quite different from the perceptions of a member of the majority viewing a minority. These perceptions have significant influences on the atmosphere in which research questions are formulated and on the conceptual, ethical, and methodological bases of research. Just as it has encouraged careers for minorities in mental health service delivery, the NIMH is providing resources for the research career development of minorities. These efforts have been undertaken not only as a matter of equity, but also as a practical necessity in mobilizing an underutilized source of talent.

Rigor in Research: "Hard" vs. "Soft" Science

During this period of realignment within the field, there have been increasing economic pressures throughout the society. It is obvious on Capitol Hill and in the funding agencies that a return to the halcyon years of the 1950s and 1960s is not imminent. Applications are evaluated more stringently, and grants have become harder to get. "Rigorousness" has become a major criterion, defined in terms of the design of a project and the extent to which results can be quantified and replicated.

Some believe, incorrectly, that the greater emphasis on rigor rules out the likelihood of support for research that cannot be scanned, stained, or centrifuged. While it is likely that important gains will be realized from the neuroscientific sphere, it would be foolhardy for the NIMH or the field to eliminate other areas from consideration. Many different scientific disciplines contribute to advances on problems that NIMH addresses. Each disorder entails a different mixture of psychological, social, and biological processes and of interactions among them. Few researchers find that their area of expertise is broad enough to answer many of the most fascinating questions about brain function or behavior, so the biomedical and behavioral sciences are increasingly entwined in interdisciplinary research. Such collaborations often foster substantial advances in the individual disciplines, as they are challenged to develop ways to assess specific aspects of brain activity or behavior without interfering with the techniques employed by the other specialties (4). Examples of this kind of research are behavioral neurochemistry studies that explore how behavior affects neurochemical events that then alter subsequent behavior. Multidisciplinary approaches are essential also in answering some vital questions about individual susceptibility to mental illness and addictions. Using these multidisciplinary approaches, investigators have shed light on the coping process and its connection to such mental illnesses as reactive depression and some forms of schizophrenia, but much remains to be learned about its neurobiological and neurophysiological concomitants. Because we do not know where the answers will be found, NIMH will maintain our effort across the board.

On the other hand, fields of study that are considered "soft," in contrast to "hard" biological research, should not be excused from meeting the standard of rigorousness. The term refers to the way scientists in any discipline frame and analyze questions, not to the nature or content of the question. There are going to be some growing pains, as recently evidenced in the debates over the scientific validity of psychoanalysis. These issues must be faced squarely so that the rich and enriching parts of the psychiatric profession and the mental health field are not discarded.

MENTAL HEALTH: THE NATIONAL AGENDA

The major challenge to the NIMH leadership is to define mental health problems in a manner that will alert the public to the seriousness of psychiatric illness and to the availability and benefits of appropriate diagnosis and treatment.

One way to approach this educational task is to examine the role of mental health in the context of specific issues and problems familiar to many people in our society. When the mental health field has taken this approach in the past, it has often made the mistake of attempting to assume responsibility for the entire problem. Only later was that perceived as naive and damaging to the credibility of the field. But where psychiatric and behavioral considerations are valid, there is a responsibility to contribute expertise to that specific part of the problem.

Five broad issues affecting people in their communities are directly relevant to the national mental health agenda. While these issues do not comprise a comprehensive listing of the mental health needs in this country, they do suggest vividly the range of tasks currently facing the mental health field.

The Homeless Who Are Mentally Ill

Homelessness is a major social issue that has reached prominence in recent years. While the mental health system cannot resolve the national problem of homelessness and homelessness per se is not a psychiatric disorder, we do know that a large, albeit unspecified, number of homeless people are mentally ill. The American Psychiatric Association's Task Force on the Homeless Mentally Ill estimated that 25 to 50 percent of the homeless suffer serious, chronic forms of mental disorders (5). An immediate need is to define the problem and identify the target population more rigorously, and research to do that is underway.

Of particular concern is the group within the homeless population who have been termed "new chronic" patients. In large part, these are young adults who are severely disabled. They are rootless and wandering. Few have ever been in institutions. The elaborate system of mental health care that has been developed in this country is, for them, a nonsystem. They may avail themselves of mental health resources during crisis episodes—or they may circulate through runaway houses or jails—but when the crisis is resolved, they revert to the streets. They have little appreciation of the concept of continuity of care.

Continuity in any context may be an alien notion to many of these young adults. Their attachments, their connectedness to family, friends, helping services, are often weak or nonexistent. It should not be surprising that they do not use the mental health system as it was designed to be used. Some service providers may perceive them as exploiting the system when they use it at all. If they do come into contact, they have a tendency to rearrange long-standing notions of how a situation ought to be handled.

These young, chronically mentally ill adults have become one of the most fundamental challenges to psychiatry. Chronicity is not a favored topic within the mental health community, and has not been historically. Morrissey and Goldman have reviewed the major reforms in the mental health care system over the past century—the mental hygiene movement and psychopathic hospitals, the child guidance movement, and the community mental health movement (6). They contend that each of these, in turn, refocused the attention of the field on prevention and treatment of acute illness, each time at the expense of the chronic patient.

Using research and demonstration grants, NIMH is beginning to develop ways to bring resources to bear more effectively on the needs of homeless people with mental illnesses and addictive disorders. Research on living arrangements outside the home for chronically disabled people, including the best combinations of psychiatric hospitals and nonhospital psychiatric care centers, is very likely to yield more information about factors that lead to appropriate care for large groups of patients. Out of this kind of research a new class of facilities for the mentally ill has been developed by combining day hospitalization and an "inn" to house day-hospital patients who require temporary residence as a transition to community living (7, 8). A basic tenet of this program is that chronically disabled patients require a system that allows easy movement between community and hospital settings. Experience with applications of this concept has demonstrated that it is possible to provide different levels of care and a range of required services within a single system.

Children and Adolescents

The quality of life experienced by this country's children and adolescents represents a second challenge and national concern to which the mental health field can contribute in discrete and potentially significant ways.

"Child mental health," as the phrase is popularly used, encompasses an array of needs and opportunities that must be addressed by the society as a whole. A major task is to define and address those elements for which mental health professionals have the necessary expertise.

There are numerous issues that warrant attention. One is depression. The fact that young children are vulnerable to clinical depression has gained wide acceptance only within the past few years; Leon Cytryn and Donald McKnew estimate that three-to-six million American children suffer depression (9). Another issue is child abuse. Although the data base is inadequate, it is well known that children are abused—sexually, psychologically, and physically—at alarming rates. Adolescent suicide is yet another critical issue. The rate of suicide among adolescents and young adults has increased 150 percent since 1960; in recent years, attention to this trend has been heightened by the phenomenon of cluster suicides that have occurred in various areas of the country.

Each of these problems has high visibility and requires expertise residing in the mental health professions. Much of the responsibility falls to the research community, and there are encouraging accomplishments. For example, Maria Kovacs has reported on a major, longitudinal study of depressive disorders in children. She noted that research in this particular area is becoming increasingly empirical, emphasizing standardized clinical assessment, diagnosis by means of operational criteria, and rigorous methodology (10).

Similarly sophisticated research is needed on the sequelae of psychological trauma experienced by children. An example is seen in Lenore Terr's follow-up studies of the children kidnapped from a Chowchilla, California, school bus and buried alive for some sixteen hours before escaping. Her findings refute the notion that children respond more flexibly than do adults to a psychic trauma. The study is of direct relevance to those who are providing mental health services to children (11).

With regard to suicide, research on risk factors would appear to be of the greatest immediate utility. At the clinical level, even gross indicators of risk will be employed by the skilled clinician as useful signposts to questions and decisions. We are looking at broad categories of risk: sociodemographic, psychological, biological, and genetic. But as Norman Farberow has noted, although the odds can only be estimated, these do determine the amount of attention given to the person being evaluated (12).

The Elderly

The elderly represent another focal point for mental health concerns. Dire warnings are constant about the "graying" of America and about the projected doubling of the 65-and-over population during the next half-century.

What gets lost in the warnings is that at any given time, only some 5 percent of all older people are in institutional settings. The remaining 95 percent are coping, often thriving, in their homes and communities. Obviously, some aspects of the aging process are difficult—for example, diminished physical capacities and mobility experienced by some people; separation from and loss of friends and family members; stresses associated with unforeseen economic constraints. Some of these changes may escalate into serious mental health problems for certain individuals, but we should not expect to treat or to resolve all of these difficulties. The mental health field can be much more effective if the major problems are targeted.

The dementias, and particularly Alzheimer's disease, have benefited from a dramatic increase in research attention in recent years. Much of this has focused on the basic processes of the illness, but greater emphasis on assessment and diagnosis, on clinical management, and on the types of supports needed by family members are also emerging.

The extent to which depression may be masked as dementia has been uncovered only recently. Depression is amenable to treatment, but only if it is diagnosed accurately. This suggests the need for more aggressive physician education and better linkages between the health and mental health care systems. General health care personnel, as well as mental health specialists, have been accused at times of harboring an attitude of "therapeutic nihilism" toward the elderly. Research that yields more effective treatments will certainly confront this attitude, but so will the provision of existing information to providers.

Violence

A final issue is violence. It is pervasive in our society. Few people have been untouched by serious, personal crime—murder, rape, assault. Public response to the Bernard Goetz subway incident in New York illustrates only the tip of the anxiety, the frustration, the anger that the constant threat of violence has spawned.

Substance-abuse disorders contribute significantly to criminal behavior, as evidenced in the high proportion of alcohol-related murders and child batterings. Suicide, particularly among the young, is a chilling indicator of the extent to which violence has become part of our culture, not only as a threat, but as a solution.

The research needs are enormous, covering the span of our knowledge base. There is, of course, interest in the question of biological bases of violence. For example, work conducted by Asberg and colleagues in Sweden and by investigators at NIMH suggests a link between metabolic products of serotonin (5-hydroxyindoleacetic acid, or 5-HIAA) and low impulse control, histories of aggression, and suicidal behavior (13). But every discipline and branch of psychiatric knowledge has much to contribute.

There is a pressing need to be concerned about the numerous ways in which mental illness intersects with violence, with criminality, and with inappropriate uses of the criminal justice system. It is well known that in many areas of the country, deinstitutionalized chronic mental patients are at a much higher than average risk for being victims of crime and that increasing numbers of mentally ill patients are being shifted into the criminal justice system. Inadequate community care facilities, a reluctance on the part of many emergency room psychiatrists to admit chronically mentally ill people who are acutely decompensated, and stringent guards against involuntary hospitalization combine to funnel many patients into jails and prisons. This process cannot be shut off by edict. But, while attempts are being made to resolve the core problem, there is much that can be done about the effects of it. The availability and quality of mental health services in jails must be improved. There is growing recognition, articulated by H. Richard Lamb and others, that psychiatry needs to take a stand for involuntary treatment; it must be pointed out that deinstitutionalization is not for everyone (14).

Research Priorities

In-house reviews of the NIMH research portfolio and reviews by prominent scientists and mental health constituent groups have made it clear that we must continue and strengthen our programs on the major disorders, particularly schizophrenia. Affective illnesses are pervasive and costly to the nation, but tremendous progress has been made in defining them and in developing treatments. It would appear that there is good reason to be optimistic about closing in on the etiology of the disorders, and our effort in this area will be maintained.

Schizophrenia
This level of accomplishment is not evident in research on schizophrenia. But rather than be discouraged by the state of

our knowledge, we need to redouble our efforts. If the NIMH does not attend to this disorder, or these disorders, who will? Resource requirements for what needs to be done are tremendous. The same level of excitement and scientific confidence that allowed this nation to mount its space program two decades ago is needed in this research domain. We need to identify the best talent in mental health research and facilitate an all-out scientific assault.

Within schizophrenia research, one of the most pressing needs is for an improved understanding of the long-term care needs of patients suffering schizophrenic disorders. In the 1960s, research demonstrated that many of the "negative" symptoms of schizophrenia—that is, underactivity, poverty of speech and affect, social withdrawal—resulted, in part, from the form of care offered to most patients: institutional management, with little active treatment. This finding provided an important impetus for the shift toward community-based care.

A decade later, research showed that the reactivity of schizophrenic patients to environmental events was not limited to the effects of understimulation; the converse was equally influential. Studies showed that social interactions, the demands of jobs, and other stimuli were equally damaging to many patients. It became evident that these patients functioned most successfully within a narrow band of social stimulation: An excess often led to relapse and a paucity, to withdrawal and clinical poverty. More research attention must be devoted to the service needs that are indicated by these clinical findings.

Prevention Research

Although the mental health field is making strides in developing a capacity to anticipate, intervene, and possibly prevent certain forms of distress, we cannot prevent the major disorders. We can, however, in certain circumstances, prevent episodes of some psychiatric illness. For example, there is intriguing evidence suggesting that appropriate family involvement in post-discharge care of patients with schizophrenia can contribute to a reduction in relapse rates. We must continue to pursue these and other important leads. The NIMH will be playing significant roles in supporting these promising lines of research, in reconceptualizing our objectives in prevention, and in refining our existing capacities.

MENTAL HEALTH SERVICES: THE NIMH ROLE

When the Omnibus Budget Reconciliation Act was enacted in 1981, the law turned over to the states authority and responsibility for numerous domestic service programs. These previously had been administered by the federal government by means of categorical grants. More than twenty-five programs, including community mental health, were consolidated into four or five block grants. These were distributed among the states on the basis of previous funding history, population, and other factors.

Relieved of CMHC support responsibilities, the NIMH budget was approximately halved, with an equivalent reduction in staff. Many people viewed this as the end, not only of the NIMH, but of the entire system of community mental health programs. This is clearly not the case. The NIMH continues to be involved directly in administration of the block grants. Lead responsibility for administering the alcohol, drug abuse, and mental health grant rests with ADAMHA, that is, at the agency level. Working with the agency, the NIMH has responsibility for reviewing annual applications and reports; participating in state compliance reviews; preparing the requisite congressional reports on the status of the program; and developing the regulations, policies, and procedures that keep this program running smoothly.

National Leadership Role

Disengagement of the federal government from all involvement in service delivery was never, in fact, an intent of the law. Immediately upon passage of the act, the ADAMHA and the NIMH began to define and to implement what has been termed the "national leadership role." This is an active rather than reactive role, demonstrated through an effective working relationship with the mental health care system and through the research priorities of the Institute. The areas noted earlier—the young adult chronically mentally ill patient, adolescent suicide, mental health needs of the elderly—did not develop in a vacuum. They are a direct response to demands that we see being placed upon providers. The general guiding principle for all of the Institute's research is that the knowledge we generate is only as good as the extent to which it relates to services. The

NIMH is evaluating continuously the relevance of our research to the needs of the mental health service delivery system and the needs of people who are mentally ill.

One example illustrating the NIMH national leadership role is the work done over the last decade, through interaction with states, to develop and assist in refining the Community Support Program. Every state now has established some form of community support system approach, and a number are interested in restructuring their service systems around that model.

The NIMH national leadership role has been essential with respect to the complexities of mental health economics today. The Institute has developed a good working relationship with the Health Care Financing Administration (HCFA), and together we have tackled some tough questions, such as the standards used to determine disability due to mental impairment under Social Security Disability Insurance. Now, of course, considerations regarding mental health care and clinical research under the diagnosis-related group (DRG) system are of increasing importance.

The NIMH is employing its national leadership role in developing comprehensive strategies to address the mental health consequences for those already affected by the acquired immune deficiency syndrome (AIDS) and to reduce the spread of AIDS among high-risk populations. NIMH activities focus on the psychiatric, behavioral and psychosocial aspects of AIDS and target high-risk populations, primarily those in the homosexual community, in regard to their concerns about AIDS, the concerns of their families and associates, and the concerns of health care providers, employers, and the general public.

Research conducted by psychiatrist Jimmie Holland at the Memorial Sloan—Kettering Cancer Center and supported by the Institute has already yielded evidence that neurological complications result from the presence of the HTLV-III virus in the spinal cord and brain. This brings a new dimension to the care of patients with AIDS and AIDS-related conditions. Clinicians must not only monitor both these groups for emotional stress—especially depression—in adapting to a highly fatal disease; they must also be on the alert for signs of mental dysfunction (15). NIMH is encouraging research to focus on links between emotional factors and immune response, as well as psychological reactions to receiving a positive result on the HTLV-III blood test. It is anticipated that studies will focus on stress factors related to the blood test to identify the HTLV-III virus in blood donors and high-risk populations. The AIDS patient, like patients with other life-threatening illnesses, struggles with the fear of imminent death, the necessity for abrupt closure on future plans, and the challenge to maintain a purpose. Knowledge of these factors is necessary to develop effective intervention strategies. In addition, there will be continuing need for public education as more specific information on AIDS becomes available.

A need presently exists to develop comprehensive AIDS-related programs in medical schools and other major teaching institutions to address the special mental health educational needs of medical students, primary-care residents, psychiatry residents, nurses, social workers, psychologists, and staff physicians; also needed are programs of training for health care workers currently providing or administratively responsible for health care to AIDS patients in community, city, county, and state hospitals, as well as clinics in community mental health centers. The goal of this NIMH initiative is to develop a comprehensive approach for the education of health care providers and trainees in the medical/psychiatric complications of AIDS, as well as in the psychosocial, psychological, and prevention-related behavioral aspects.

CONCLUSION

Over the last four decades, the NIMH has played a strategic role in the development of the entire spectrum of the mental health field. In the Institute's own laboratories and in research facilities throughout the country and the world, thousands of investigators under the auspices of NIMH have been at work on problems that span the full range of biomedical and behavioral disciplines. Research supported by the NIMH has led to a substantial increase in information about the causes, treatment, and prevention of mental illnesses and the factors that help foster mental health. The NIMH is committed to mobilizing the best possible intellectual, technical, and moral resources over a wide range of knowledge and perspectives not only to sustain the tradition it has established, but also to address appropriately the challenges still before us.

REFERENCES

1. Mukheryee, S., Shukla, S., & Woodle, J. (1983). Misdiagnosis of schizophrenia in bipolar patients: A multiethnic comparison. *American Journal of Psychiatry, 140,* 1571–1574.
2. Lawson, W. B. (in press). Chronic mental illness and the black family. *American Journal of Social Psychiatry.*
3. Adebimpe, V. R. (1981). White norms and psychiatric diagnosis of black patients. *American Journal of Psychiatry, 138,* 279–285.
4. Institute of Medicine. (1984). *Research on mental illness and addictive disorders—Progress and prospects.* Washington, DC: National Academy Press, 1984.
5. Lamb. H. R. (Ed.). (1984). *The homeless mentally ill.* Washington, DC: The American Psychiatric Association.
6. Morrissey, J. P., & Goldman, H. H. (1984). Cycles of reform in the care of the chronically mentally ill. *Hospital and Community Psychiatry, 35,* 785.
7. Gudeman, J. E., Shore, M. F., & Dickey, B. (1983). Day hospitalization and an inn instead of inpatient care of psychiatric patients. *New England Journal of Medicine, 308,* 749–753.
8. Gudeman, J. E., & Shore, M. F. (1984). Beyond deinstitutionalization: A new class of facilities for the mentally ill. *New England Journal of Medicine, 311,* 832–836.
9. McKnew, D., & Cytryn, L. (1983). *Why isn't Johnny crying? Coping with depression with children* New York: Norton.
10. Kovacs, M., Feinberg, T. A., Crouse-Novak, M. A., et al. (1984). Depressive disorders in childhood. *Archives of General Psychiatry, 4,* 229–237 and 643–649.
11. Terr, L. (1983). Chowchilla revised: The effects of psychic trauma four years after a school bus kidnapping. *American Journal of Psychiatry, 140,* 1543–1550.
12. Farberow, N. (1984). Youth suicide. *Psychiatric News, 19* (7), 54–55.
13. Asberg, M., Thoren, P., & Traskman, L. (1976). Seratonin depression—A biochemical subgroup within the affective disorders. *Science, 191,* 478–480.
14. Lamb, H. R. (1984). Commentary: Keeping the mentally ill out of jail. *Hospital and Community Psychiatry, 35,* 529.
15. Holland, J. C. (1985). AIDS impairs mental functions. *ADAMHA News, 11*(8):1.

4

The Economics of Mental Health Care in a Changing Economic and Health Care Environment

Richard M. Scheffler

Even the most casual follower of the health care system in the United States is aware of the increasingly rapid pace of change. Not since the watershed legislation of almost twenty years ago, when Medicare and Medicaid were passed, have both the federal and state governments been so active in stimulating change. Most of the basic changes center around the notion that the health care system has grown without control, has no built-in mechanism to level off its rate of expansion, and is inefficient in the sense that it may not be giving the public its money's worth. Within this context, the mental health delivery system—if it can really be thought of as a system—is being impacted by the overall changes in the health care delivery system. This chapter will sketch out the major thrusts and nature of changes now beginning since the passage of the TEFRA legislation, diagnosis-related groups (DRGs), and competition in health. Within this context, some of the potential impacts on delivery of mental health care will be addressed. Finally, a few thoughts are presented about the problems being created and where things may be headed in the mental health area.

THE FORCES OF CHANGE

In the early 1970s, I left the University of North Carolina–Chapel Hill to spend some time in Washington, D.C., at the Institute of Medicine. There I observed federal health policy being made and the impact of various lobbying groups. Among the lessons I learned was that change in this environment would not happen without a major crisis. The parties involved in health policy, including the feds, the professional organizations, consumer groups, insurance companies, the private sector, and organized labor, were quite content to live with the status quo. Most of the concern centered around the rising cost of health care and how it could be financed. Even with early cost increases of 12–15 percent, changes were not possible. For the most part, the major activity did not have enough to gain to justify the uncertainty of change.

By the time I left Washington, D.C. in 1980, a somewhat new level of concern about the rising cost of health care had emerged. The rising cost of health care was being seen as one of the major factors increasing the federal deficit as well as state deficits. These deficits were linked to higher interest rates and to higher taxes. It was now being recognized that the growth of health care expenditures was an important factor in the overall growth and health of the economy as a whole and state economies as well. After all, 40 percent of hospital costs and about 20 percent of physician costs are federally financed. In addition, the fastest growing part of the health system—long-term care— is financed by Medicaid. In the minds of some government leaders, health care costs had now reached the point of being a potential threat to the ability of the economy to grow, whereas in the previous decade the growth of the economy had been seen as a limiting factor in the growth of the health care sector.

At the state level, budget deficits also stimulated changes. In California, the budget deficit projection in 1981 and 1982 led to major changes in the Medicaid system—competitive bidding for

Medicaid patients by hospitals, as well as legislation to allow the growth of preferred provider organizations. States across the country made major changes in their health care financing that are currently being studied but whose impact is not well known or understood at this date.

THRUSTS OF CHANGE

The major thrust of change in health care centers around the notion of competition. It is useful to understand that the health care system was not selected or singled out to be left open to changes and forces evoked by competition. Although the Reagan administration had a lot to do with encouraging the competitive model and deregulating the health care system and the economy as a whole, it was following a trend that can be traced to previous administrations. Under President Carter, a bill sponsored by Senator Edward Kennedy was passed to deregulate the airline industry, and measures were taken to remove trade barriers. It is more useful to view the trend toward competition in health care as part of the overall trend in our economic system, spanning both political parties, toward less regulation.

DRGs, which prospectively pay hospitals a fixed rate per type of admission, are perhaps the most significant health policy change in the last twenty years. Although they are still being phased in, their impact is already being observed. Hospital lengths of stay are down, as are hospital costs. Neither of these impacts is large at this time, but the direction of the impact appears clear. The impact on the mental health area is unknown as of yet because many hospitals opted out of the DRG plan, as they are allowed to until a more appropriate method of categorizing mental health is developed. Other issues in the DRG plan need to be resolved as well: (1) How will capital improvements be included? (2) How will technological change be financed? (3) What will happen to the cost of medical education? Indeed, DRGs are changing the structure of the hospital industry.

Another major thrust of change is in the organization and financing of outpatient care. Preferred provider organizations (PPOs) are the most interesting new delivery model. In effect, PPOs are really only an alternative method of paying for mental

health care that may or may not have much of an impact on the
delivery of care and organization of the mental health system.
The most common forms of PPOs are being organized by insurers such as Blue Cross or Blue Shield. They select or ask providers in an area to discount their fees for health care and in return
promise access to their patient population. In areas with a large
supply of providers, this inducement is quite powerful. To the
patient population, the PPO option is offered at a reduced premium but restricts the use of services to those providers in the
PPO plan. A patient who uses an out-of-plan provider must bear
a majority of, if not all, costs. Finally, providers in general will
continue to be paid on a fee-for-service basis, albeit at a discounted fee.

THE IMPACT OF ECONOMIC CHANGE

Although I am not aware of a study that forecasts the growth of
mental health care in the United States, I am aware of a few
trends that help paint a design that may be useful for discussion
purposes. The most systemic is a demographic one. The baby-
boom generation is approaching middle age. It is well known
that the use of mental health care is highest in the middle-aged
group. At the same time, the overall population is aging, with
significant increases in the over-65 age group now apparent.
Moreover, the rate of increase of those over 80 or 85 is also increasing rapidly. It is well known that a significant proportion
of long-term institutional care involves the delivery of mental
health care. Data suggest that 20 percent of expenditures in
nursing homes, the fastest growing component of the health
care system, are for mental health services. Improved diagnostic
data may even increase this estimate. In addition, a large share
of mental health care of the aged is being borne by family
members who may increasingly resist providing this care as it
strains their own family ties. In sum, the demographics suggest
an increased need for mental health care.

As is usually the case, economics usually determines whether
this need will be translated into economic demand for services.
As we mentioned earlier, the overall thrust of change in the
delivery of health care and mental health services is one motivated by cost savings. Health care insurers, the government, and
large purchasers of mental health care, such as corporations,

still remain uncomfortable with mental health services. Except as regards violence from untreated persons, and perhaps drug and alcohol addiction, these groups do not understand or care about the potential value of mental health care. This situation is not new.

What is new is that under competitive pressures the value of mental health care is being increasingly scrutinized. Insurers and states are increasing the limits placed on mental health profits. Limitations on inpatient care (e.g., 30 days) and out-patient care (e.g., 50 visits) are not uncommon; neither are lifetime limits on expenditures (e.g., $50,000). Further controls include the increased use of co-payments and deductibles. My own study of the Federal Health Benefits Plan—Blue Cross/Blue Shield option has demonstrated how increases in co-payments can alter the amount of mental health care, as well as the type of care (inpatient vs. outpatient), delivered. Most studies show that patients respond to price (out-of-pocket) increases and reduce their use of services. Furthermore, given equivalent increases in out-of-pocket costs, they are more likely to reduce mental health than physical health care. The message here appears to be that competition and cost increase caused by benefit changes may have a significant impact on the use of mental health care.

The most expensive item in the delivery of mental health care is clearly inpatient care, with the small percentage of inpatients accounting for a very large share of the costs. Firm estimates are lacking for the system as a whole, but data on specific health insurance plans show that 4–5 percent of the inpatient users may account for 20–40 percent of the costs. The uncertainty involved in bearing this type of risk makes insurers uncomfort-able about open-ended benefit packages for mental health ser-vice. It would appear that changes underway which reduce benefit coverages for inpatient care will increase the use of county hospitals, which have been the place of last resort for mental health care.

DRGs, soon to be put into effect in the hospital system for mental health services, will further pressure the delivery of care. Although the categories for DRG reimbursement are still being developed, it can be safely said that they will be inadequate. The severity of mental illness and the costs required for treatment in a hospital—especially length of stay—will be extremely difficult to factor in any set of DRG categories. Whatever the categories chosen, healthier patients will be preferred to sicker ones, especially for financially distressed hospitals, because they cost less to treat; thus the difference between the prospective rate the hospital will receive and its costs will be the greatest. However, it is important to note that DRGs will not have a really significant impact on inpatient mental health use until they are used by states in their Medicaid payment system. Additional impacts will be felt when private payers (insurance companies) begin to adopt the DRG system, in part to avoid the transfer of hospital costs to them from Medicare and Medicaid. The response of states and insurance companies to DRGs is quite varied and complex. Clearly we need to watch this development quite closely.

CONCLUSIONS

Budget deficits for the U.S. Treasury, as well as many state treasuries, over the last five years have produced the mandate for change in the health care system and, in effect, the mental health care system. The excess supply of providers has increased competition, as has the deregulation of the health care system. Short-run cost savings appear to dominate the motivation for change.

It appears that the system-wide changes impacting on the health care delivery system, such as prospective hospital reimbursement (DRGs) and preferred provider organizations (PPOs), will change rules governing the future of the delivery of mental health care. Mental health providers and policy makers will likely be watching the impact of these changes on physical health care as an important indicator of the potential impact on mental health care. To date, the preliminary evidence suggests that DRGs cause lower lengths of hospital stay and perhaps lower rates of admissions. It is too early to have even preliminary results on PPOs. However, it is clear that physicians are joining in many areas of the country and discounting their fees in the 20–30 percent range.

It appears to me that mental health policy makers as well as providers can have a significant impact on their fate. One way of doing that is to get more involved in defining the appropriate level of mental health treatment. Related to this is the increased use of utilization review (UR) to control any inappropriate delivery of mental health care, especially in hospitals. Cost savings that could result in high-quality UR may increase the overall use of appropriate mental health care.

Recent evidence points clearly to cost saving by health maintenance organizations (HMOs) in the delivery of mental health care. The outpatient HMO cost of mental health care in one study was 2/3 as high as a fee-for-service system in the same area. The order of magnitude does not really matter. The message appears to be that organized mental health care systems with appropriate UR could be the direction in which delivery is heading.

It still remains unclear whether the growth of HMO-type delivery of mental health care will parallel that of physical health care. Integration of service and cost offsets (the cost of mental health care being lower than the cost of physical health care), if they exist, support this model. The alternative of a mental health HMO, or one that has contractual arrangements with various HMOs, may be a promising model. Some are beginning to emerge, and their success or failure should be closely watched.

REFERENCES

Horgan, C. (1984). *The demand for ambulatory mental health services from specialty providers.* Unpublished manuscript.

Keeler, E. B., Rolph, J., Duan, N., Hanley, J., & Manning, W. Jr. (1982). *The demand for episodes of medical treatment: Interim results from the health insurance experiment* (R-2829-HHS). Santa Monica, CA: Rand Corporation.

Manning, W., & Weik, K. (1984). *Preliminary results of a controlled trial of the effect of a prepayment group practice on the outpatient use of mental health service* (WD-2361-NIMH). Santa Monica, CA: Rand Corporation.

Manning, W., Duan, N., Newhouse, J. P., Wells, K. B., & Ware, J. E. (in press). Cost sharing and the use of ambulatory mental health services. *American Psychologist.*

McGuire, T. G. (1984). *Financing psychotherapy.* Cambridge: Ballinger Publishing.

Taube, C., Lee, E. S., & Forthofer, R. N. (1984). DRGs in psychiatry: An empirical evaluation. *Medical Care, 22,* 597.

Trauner, J. (1983). *Preferred provider organization: The California experiment.* San Francisco, University of California, Institute for Health Policy Studies.

Watts, C. A., & Scheffler, R. M. Demand for outpatient mental health services in a heavily insured population: The case of Blue Cross/Blue Shield federal employees health benefits plan. Unpublished manuscript.

5

The Guilds:
An Organizational Analysis

Charles A. Kiesler

This chapter focuses on the major guilds of mental health, the problems they solve, and the problems they create. In this analysis, I will bring to bear some of my own research interests in national mental health policy, my previous experience in Washington as executive officer of the American Psychological Association, and my substantive background as a social psychologist with an interest in organizations, power, and interpersonal influence. I will argue that one's training and one's organizational involvement almost inevitably produce a biased perspective that inhibits knowledge acquisition and use, impedes dispassionate problem definition, and leads to a narrow focus on national policy. As a psychologist, I have my own perspective, background, and biases, but I will struggle to be as even-handed as possible. However, total objectivity in human thought and judgment is realized only imperfectly at best.

In our discussion, we will focus mainly upon the American Psychological Association and the American Psychiatric Association as the main representatives of their fields. We do so not because they are the only important ones (they are not) but because they tend to dominate public policy. Most of our re-marks could be applied to almost any guild within the mental health field. We will focus on guilds as organizations per se, composed of true believers, biased perceivers, and implicit theorists about human behavior. We will look at the im-plications of some of these issues for the problems facing the mental health field in the future and for the issues that need to be faced in order to enhance public policy evaluation and change.

GUILDS AS ORGANIZATIONS

Mental health professional guilds are organizations that have certain advantages and disadvantages irrespective of the pro-fessional core or intent of the organization. Mental health professional guilds are important because they represent and coordinate the overall aggregate policies and practices in the United States regarding mental health. However, they are also organizations and, as such, have certain properties independent of their professional knowledge base. Let us discuss some of these organizational properties and their implications.

Professional organizations have power. And with that power comes a sense of importance that makes it very tempting to use the power as a form of positive self-evaluation.

Professional organizations become vehicles for career ad-vancement. People advance in the organization only if others notice them. Thus, certain kinds of attention-getting behaviors are practiced within organizations irrespective of whether they are public spirited or contribute to the long-term goals of the organization. Some issues get discussed and some perspectives get taken that can be predicted solely on the basis of how individuals get attention in large organizations.

Organizations promote consensual views. Any organization or social group is under implicit social pressures to adopt common views and to think similarly about issues important to the organization. The degree to which this is true is a function of the number of people in the organization, the importance of the organization for the individual, and the importance of the topic for the organization (cf. Kiesler & Kiesler, 1969). For example, Jacobs & Campbell (1961) have shown that common views developed within a particular group can continue to exist even though the original individuals have rotated out and the group is now composed of individuals who were not present when the common view was developed.

Organizations represent centrist views. Partly because of the implicit pressures to adopt common views, partly because of a consensus about the organization's development, partly because of treatment of deviants, views that deviate from the organization's official views are raised less frequently in the organizational context than they are privately by the individuals comprising the organization. Because of the biased public focus of the organization, attitudinal minorities are heard less frequently and perceived to be smaller than is in fact the case.

Organizations are slow to react. There is a common organizational lethargy that inhibits clear and dramatic action and organizational change. Bureaucratic wheels grind slowly and finely, but not necessarily rationally. I am struck by the number of issues that were hotly contested seven years ago when I headed the American Psychological Association and are still being discussed there.

Organizations resist change. Organizations resist change from the inside, but they are especially resistant to changes proposed from the outside that might affect them. It is commonly acknowledged that the American Medical Association (AMA) has, since the 1930s, resisted every major piece of social legislation potentially affecting it, including social security, Medicaid, Medicare, and most forms of national health insurance. To a social psychologist, the AMA's resistance to change is less noteworthy than the fact that many people find it surprising (or embarrassing). It is predictable, and clearly a part of human nature within organizations. Indeed, we should expect the organization to resist change even more than any individual member on such issues.

These natural organizational processes probably lead to mental health guilds' being different publicly in action, pronouncement, and reflection from any randomly drawn subgroup of individuals from them. Thus any individually drawn psychiatrist and psychologist will probably agree more on professional and public policy issues than would the two organizations representing them. However, this is not to say that psychiatrists and psychologists (or psychiatric nurses and clinical social workers) are identical. There is some evidence that clinical psychologists and psychiatrists are more alike in personality characteristics than are psychiatrists and the rest of the medical profession (Henry, Sims, & Spray, 1971). But in certain natural and expected ways they are quite different in background and perspective. It is these differences to which we now turn.

DIFFERENCES IN PERSPECTIVE

Our thesis in this section is that there are certain aspects of training and preparation (and self-selection) that would lead us to expect psychiatrists and psychologists to think differently about certain problems and issues of mental health and mental health policy. Some of these differences in perspective and thought processes are submerged in implicit assumptions about what mental health and mental health problems are. To the extent that these processes are only implicit and not explicit, they inhibit scientific progress in the field and logical discussion of national policy alternatives. Let us look at some of these differences and discuss some of their implications. In the interest of brevity, I have oversimplified the description of training in both fields, but would argue that the basic implications of the differences would hold in a more complete and qualified description.

Psychiatrists

It is obvious but not trivial that psychiatrists first and foremost are physicians who go to medical school. Medical education basically leads to a professional orientation, not a scientific one. The biological sciences are obviously a core aspect of medical education, but the students approach it more as consumers than originators of science. Further, inevitably and naturally, medical school leads to a very biological orientation toward human problems—a fact that may be less important in some specialties, such as anaesthesiology or orthopedics, than it is for psychiatry, which must deal with the whole person in a social context. In typical medical school training, there is little or nothing learned about scientific design, methodology, and the statistics and mathematics common to the scientific enterprise. Psychiatrists are trained to make good decisions based on diagnostic evidence, and they practice inductive reasoning based on previous case experience (as opposed to the deductive style common, but not universal, in science). Psychiatric residencies are typically in teaching hospitals. In them, one is more likely to see psychotics than neurotics. As a result of those experiences, one might expect psychiatrists to see mental health more as a medical problem and to be concerned about issues of legal liability. It is our thesis that the general biological context of training in psychiatry, and the array of cases that one might be expected to see in a psychiatric residency in a first-rate teaching hospital, would lead one to have certain expectations and a biased perspective about the patient population (and even about the underlying causes and prognosis of a given case).

Psychologists

There are really two brands of psychologists that one might discuss here. About half of the American Psychological Association is composed of psychologists who regard themselves as scientific psychologists (I am one of those). Their training is heavily mathematical, methodological, and statistical in nature. They are very skeptical, sometimes (it seems) about almost everything. Philosophers of science such as Feyerabend see them as the most overtly scientific group in the many scientific fields, striving to make implicit assumptions explicit, detailing hypothetical relationships among theoretical variables, and attempting to theorize very explicitly about human behavior. A typical approach to a new research area is to strive to get an increasingly narrow but deep focus on the area—to make more precise predictions about an increasingly constrained area of discussion. Certain approaches to problems are commonly conceived to be fruitless, because of their checkered history in psychology. One such problem of importance to mental health professionals is that of typologies. Categorizing groups of people is usually seen to be a fruitless and error-prone exercise by scientific psychologists.

Most clinical psychologists have undergone a good deal of this scientific training. In most graduate programs of psychology, budding clinical psychologists are obligated to take core courses in statistics and scientific design, obligated to do a masters thesis and a dissertation that will occupy most of two years of their graduate careers, and often deprecated for any desire to help other people. They come out of this with a "healthy" scientific skepticism; they distrust typologies greatly; they have considerably less clinical experience than psychiatrists, particularly in a hospital setting and with patients who have major psychoses; they are very oriented toward the understanding of normal human behavior, with less orientation toward and experience with the seriously disturbed. They are very likely to see mental health issues as primarily reflecting cognitive or behavioral problems or some combination of them.

The above description pertains more to the products of graduate programs that identify themselves with the Boulder model. More recently, there has been a literal explosion of professional schools of psychology with a different orientation. The graduates of these schools tend to have more clinical experience and less scientific training than their colleagues from more traditionally oriented programs. Their de-emphasis on scientific training and emphasis on clinical training should in those respects produce a perspective more like psychiatrists. However, a major difference still remains—a lack of a biological orientation to the major problems of mental health.

Implications for Treatment

We have oversimplified our description of the training of psychiatrists and psychologists to make a point. There are differences in their training, and the differences are not trivial. The differences in training lead to some different perspectives on problems facing the mental health field. Consider some of the implications of the following assumptions for how national mental health problems should be handled:

1. If the basic mental health problem is medical, then surely psychiatrists should be in charge of the field and the individual cases.

2. If the treatment is in a hospital (or could lead to hospitalization), then psychiatrists perhaps should be in charge (partly because of expertise and partly because of legal liability).

3. If the problem is cognitive or behavioral, then psychologists know more about these variables.

4. If the basic issue for a particular case or field is one of interpreting scientific evidence, then psychologists may be better prepared to do that.

We are not claiming that any of these assumptions are valid. Rather, we are saying that the variation of assumptions can lead to quite different conclusions about the proper way to go about solving problems in mental health. In essence, both fields are caught in a web of their own training and *Zeitgeist*. For example, the re-medicalization of psychiatry can in this context be seen as an attempt to define mental health problems as problems of medicine. If psychiatrists are physicians, and if the basic problems in mental health are medical in nature, then enhanced medical training can only lead to enhanced performance. The controversial use of the term "medical psychotherapy" is a very natural extension of this line of thinking. However, the above discussion of the preparation of psychologists could be used to predict their quite angry response to the use of that term.

Further, various attempts to keep psychologists out of Medicare, Medicaid, Blue Cross/Blue Shield plans, and other private plans can be seen as a logical extension of the notion that these problems are basically medical in nature. I know that some psychologists say that this conflict is basically economic in nature. On the other hand, my experience with psychiatrists leads me to think that it is more than simply an economic issue. Many of them believe—because of their medical orientation and implicit beliefs about the causes of mental health problems— that it is dangerous to let psychologists go unsupervised.

From their different preparation and perspectives, it could be predicted that psychiatrists and psychologists would have quite different attitudes about Diagnostic and Statistical Manual DSM III and any other taxonomy of medical diagnosis applied to mental health problems. Such taxonomies in general have a much more positive history and reputation in medicine than in psychology. Psychologists are not only skeptical, but cynical, about DSM III. They feel it is internally consistent, but does not fit the real world, and that its major purpose is not to fit the needs of the patient, but the needs of third-party payers.

Psychiatrists and psychologists, because of their training, can be expected to think quite differently about mental health problems quite often. Not all of this is due simply to training. There surely is some self-selection leading an individual to choose one career or the other because the type of implicit explanation— biological versus psychological—is somehow more appealing to them. Each group has a biased set of experiences and therefore a biased perspective. This biased perspective is due partly to training and partly to self-selection, but there is also a set of experiences obtained that reinforces the bias. It is commonly acknowledged, for example, that patients sort themselves out. Individual therapists are not dealing with randomly drawn sets of problems. Parents of a hallucinating child might be more likely to take that child to a psychiatrist, because they see the problem as potentially biological in nature. Parents of a child with serious behavior problems in school might perhaps take their child to a psychologist, because they see the problem as behavioral in nature. Since the style of practice in both fields is essentially reactive—the helping professionals tend to wait in their offices for problems to come to them—it is difficult for them to maintain awareness of the self-selection of those problems prior to their contact.

Neither set of professionals sees a random set of all kinds of problems. Bandura (1978) makes the point that it is only the failures that the therapists see, rather than a randomly drawn subset of people with a particular type of problem. He says, "the disadvantaged, ineffectual, and powerless members of the various diagnostic categories . . . serve as the major source of data for theories of psychopathology because researchers lack access to most of the successful schizophrenics, the successful depressives, and the successful compulsives. Rather, we admire their paintings, enjoy their music, read their novels, and vote for them in public office. Textbooks that catalogue the characteristic infirmities of the different psychopathologies rarely, if ever, cite examples of the afflicted who succeed, such as the Lincolns among the depressed." (p. 95).

Consequently each type of professional brings a certain biased perspective to the problem, sees a biased sample of patients (who themselves to some extent select whom they are going to see), and as well sees only a biased sample of the diagnostic categories (i.e., the failures). Further, both sets of professionals see a biased sample of the patients' behavior. That is to say, neither group tends to see patients in their natural environments but only in the "role" of patient.

Common Biases of Perspective

The above discussion leads to some sense of what might be expected to be somewhat different but biased perspectives on the part of psychologists and psychiatrists. These biases in perspective, we have argued, would be naturally expected to surface within the respective guilds, to be conservatively represented there, and to lead in turn to an even greater difference in perspective as publicly represented through the guild mechanism.

There are also some commonalities in perspective, both advantageous and disadvantageous. In both fields, clinical training can be seen as experiential in nature and based on role models. Clinical experience is a worthwhile and important ingredient of preparation to handle mental health problems. One would not advocate otherwise. On the other hand, there are certain drawbacks to the process of gaining clinical experience in training. To the extent that it is experiential in nature, it is subject to the common flaws in human thought processes that make difficult a one-to-one correspondence between the real world and one's perception of it. There is an imperfect feedback loop between clinical judgment, the complex stimulus array on which it is based, and the outcomes of clinical judgment on the patient. Experience leads one to be an imperfect learner from a complex environment. Partly because the cues and feedback loops are somewhat ambiguous in nature, one can develop great confidence about one's human judgmental capacities that may be quite independent of fact.

The process of learning through role models—a critical ingredient of the professional training in both fields—has similar limitations. The process of professional role modeling also carries with it an ingredient of imitation, rather than skepticism and questioning. Since the professional behaviors being modeled are themselves very complex and imperfectly understood, it is only natural that the imitation of them would be even more imperfect. Phrased a different way, and in extreme form, if everything we were doing in the treatment of mental patients in the United States was wrong at some level, our treatment practice would still be extremely difficult to change because of the ways we train treatment providers. I would argue that both groups could use more healthy skepticism about the validity of their own feelings, perceptions, and guesses regarding mental health problems.

As a result of these processes, mental health treatment providers of both professions are probably enticed to believe that they have a greater level of understanding of mental health problems than they in fact do. Thus, it is very difficult for them to try metaphorically to stand aside from their training to question the whole system of service provision. To some extent it is very difficult to look at the whole national system and to discuss how the total system might be differently implemented. (Trying to inspect the implications of alternative total systems is a desirable practice in policy analysis.) Instead one is enticed more toward a perspective of looking at professional life at the margin (to use the economists' term), to say what we have been doing in the past and how we might do it a little better in the future. The prospect of breaking with the past—to consider potentially radical departures from current practices and outcome—is difficult to accomplish with the systems and organizations that we are naturally tied to. Guilds play a central role in this system, with all of their positive features and natural drawbacks.

IN THE PUBLIC INTEREST

Top-down Policy Analysis

Elsewhere, I have discussed an approach to public policy evaluation and analysis in mental health, which I call "top-down analysis" to distinguish it from bottom-up analysis (Kiesler, 1983). Bottom-up analysis, as I define it, is the approach we generally use in the field of mental health. Using this approach, we inspect what we have done in the past and attempt to enhance it or improve it for the future. In this context we would look at patients treated, improved technologies, increased financial commitments for treatment and research, improved training of professionals, and the like. All of these are valued outcomes for improvement of mental health services and treatment, and I certainly do not argue that they are in any sense to be deprecated.

I do argue, however, that when one only looks bottom-up—looking at improvements at the margin in the system of service, or in providers, or in number of patients treated—there are very significant elements of national mental health policy that go unexamined. Consequently, in addition to this bottom-up analysis I also advocate a top-down analysis, which does not substitute for, but rather complements, the more typical policy analysis.

In a top-down analysis we attempt to look at what the nation does in the name of mental health, whether intended or not, at what cost, to whom, and with what effectiveness (cf. Kiesler, 1980). Several startling things can come out of such a comparison of top-down with bottom-up analysis. For example, the incidence of mental health problems is sufficiently substantial in the United States that we could never hope to train enough psychiatrists and psychologists to handle all of them, using traditional treatment methods. Thus a public policy based on psychotherapy and other mental health care delivered solely by psychologists and psychiatrists could only handle a trivial proportion of the total need. Further, discussions of the effectiveness of psychotherapy pale before the fact that psychotherapy as it is traditionally carried out could only handle a minority of the people needing care, regardless of which professional group (or all professional groups) delivered the therapy (Kiesler, 1984).

Top-down analysis leads us to the conclusion that the substantial majority of the mental health dollar spent for care in the United States goes for inpatient treatment, with the effectiveness of such treatment, at least at a national level, being relatively unexamined. Recently, I and others have reviewed the evidence comparing the outcome and cost-effectiveness of inpatient care of serious mental disorders compared to a variety of forms of alternative care in the community (Kiesler, 1982; Braun et al., 1981; Straw, 1982). Alternative care is typically more effective and less expensive than hospital treatment. However, ironically, the incidence of mental hospitalization is increasing, not decreasing (Kiesler & Sibulkin, 1984). One policy issue is that there are incentives in both public and private insurance plans for mental hospitalization and against outpatient treatment. Top-down policy analysis leads us to ask which methods of mental health care are most efficacious and cost-effective.

Top-down analysis also leads us to point to certain types of issues that are totally unexplored. Consider the nation's alternative decisions about public policy and mental health. One category of decisions concerns where the public dollar should be placed. When one considers such alternatives, one is very quickly led to thoughts about funding different systems of care. To what extent, for example, should mental health care be encouraged in health maintenance organizations (HMOs)? Should such

HMO care be routinely integrated into existing HMOs, or is it worthwhile to consider HMOs concentrated on mental health care in isolation? Do community mental health centers effectively handle treatment over a broad array of cases? If so, is the effectiveness of that care sufficient to demand more public dollars than simply the cost of a case-by-case basis? (For example, financing consultation and education or bricks and mortar.)

Top-down policy analysis, as a supplement to existing bottom-up analysis, can lead to an array of important and critical questions for policy analysis. This type of question demands some conceptualization of the total public problem in order to see how specific current practices work and to consider possible alternative or supplementary public policies. To the extent that professional guilds have a biased focus that leads them to concentrate particularly on an aspect of the total problem, such top-down policy analysis is inhibited. Such policy analyses, we would argue, are in the public interest, and it is worthwhile to consider what actions guilds might take in order to enhance the promotion of the public interest.

What Must Guilds Do

As we have discussed in the preceding sections, guilds must somehow make less salient their own focus on a particular mental health problem and engage in collaborative behavior to help define the country's total problem. They must dispassionately consider potential alternative policies without first considering whether such policies are in their narrower professional interests. Consequently, guilds must acknowledge the scope of the mental health problem in the United States and seriously consider their own numerical inadequacy to deal with the total breadth of that problem. Differently phrased, the guilds must become more problem oriented and less profession oriented. This is not an easy task, and guilds need to consider how interdisciplinary, interprofessional linkages for such policy analysis might be accomplished. A basic conclusion from research on conflict reduction is the need for competing groups to develop superordinate goals (Sherif & Sherif, 1953).

There is also an active professional field regarding the policy sciences, with which psychology and psychiatry have not had great contact. Policy research and policy analysis have traditionally depended heavily on the study of economics, political science, mathematics and statistics, demography, epidemiology, and the law. Somehow both psychiatry and psychology must discover ways to promote such knowledge in their own professional training and to ease the acquisition and use of such knowledge into their own discussions.

A disproportionate share of discussion about mental health leads to discussions of treatment providers or treatment processes. Such discussions inevitably start from a flawed but not identical set of assumptions for each field. Such discussions, starting as they do from different assumptions, cannot be resolved on *a priori* grounds. I would argue that discussion should focus more on outcome of treatment, rather than treatment provider or process. What works best should be publicly supported. Both fields should promote more research on treatment outcome and agree in advance to act on the conclusions produced by such research.

Discussions of systems of delivery of service (all of which do not involve any one field, but usually combinations of them) are greatly in the public interest. There has been little or no research comparing systems of service delivery, particularly regarding outcomes of such service. A collaborative interdisciplinary effort to help provide this very complicated brand of research is greatly needed and clearly in the public interest.

Compared to other public policies, mental health policy has been very deficient in developing a proper data base for research. For example, there is considerable variation in epidemiological estimates of mental health problems, ranging from 15 to 35 percent. We also do not understand in detail how many people are hospitalized for mental disorder, the treatment received there, or the complex judgments underlying the diagnoses (primary or secondary) and the committing actions.

Finally, there has been great reluctance by both professions to face up to the issue of cost-effectiveness of treatment. Both professions seem to focus on why and how they provide good service, and both seem very skittish about trying to look at the cost-effectiveness of such care. Detailed consideration and considerable research on the complex question of the cost-effectiveness of alternative treatment strategies is greatly in the public interest and should be encouraged.

CONCLUSIONS

In this chapter we have focused on the professional guilds as organizations. We have stressed that there are certain natural aspects of organizations, which leads one to expect them to be conservative regarding actions, interests, and attitudes, and self-enhancing regarding reputation. We have described how differences in the training of psychiatrists and psychologists can lead to biased perspectives, with predictable consequences. We have tried to describe future problems in national mental health policy and how a top-down policy analysis usefully supplements the more typical analysis done in the past. Organizational change is difficult to accomplish, but we have urged that the guilds take steps leading to cooperation and coordination in the public interest.

REFERENCES

Bandura, A. (1978). On paradigms and recycled ideologies. *Cognitive Therapy and Research, 2,* 79–103.

Braun, P., Kochansky, G., Shapiro, R., Greenberg, S., Gudeman, J. E., Johnson, S., & Shore, M. F. (1981). Overview: Deinstitutionalization of psychiatric patients, a critical review of outcome studies. *American Journal of Psychiatry, 138*(6), 736–749.

Henry, W. E., Sims, J. H., & Spray, S. L. (1971). *The fifth professions: Becoming a psychotherapist.* San Francisco: Jossey-Bass.

Jacobs, R. C., & Campbell, D. J. (1961). The perpetuation of an arbitrary tradition through several generations of a laboratory microculture. *Journal of Abnormal and Social Psychology, 62,* 649–658.

Kiesler, C. A. (1980). Mental health policy as a field of inquiry for psychology. *American Psychologist, 35,* 1066–1080.

Kiesler, C. A. (1982). Mental hospitals and alternative care: Non-institutionalization as potential public policy for mental patients. *American Psychologist, 37,* 349–360.

Kiesler, C. A. (1983). Psychology and mental health policy. In M. Hersen, A. E. Kazdin, & A. S. Bellack (Eds.), *The clinical psychology handbook* (pp. 63–82). New York: Pergamon Press.

Kiesler, C. A. (1984). Psychotherapy research and top-down policy analysis. In R. L. Spitzer & J. B. Williams (Eds.), *Psychotherapy research: Where are we and where should we go?* (pp. 360–371). New York: Guilford Publications, Inc.

Kiesler, C. A., & Kiesler, S. (1969). *Conformity.* Boston: Addison-Wesley.

Kiesler, C. A., & Sibulkin, A. E. (1984). Episodic rate of mental hospitalization: Stable or increasing? *American Journal of Psychiatry, 141,* 44–48.

Sherif, M., & Sherif, C. W. (1953). *Groups in harmony and tension.* New York: Harper & Row.

Straw, R. (1982). *Meta-analysis of deinstitutionalization in mental health.* Unpublished doctoral dissertation, Northwestern University, Evanston, IL.

6

Mental Health Care in HMOs: Practice and Potential

Saul Feldman
Beth Goldman

The conventional wisdom about the future of health care in the United States forecasts glowing prospects and rapid growth for health maintenance organizations (HMOs) all across the country. While it is often tempting to be critical of such predictions, there is strong evidence to suggest they may well be correct. The growth pattern of the past few years, the national concern about the rising costs of health care, the entry into the HMO field of large for-profit organizations, the success of many HMOs, and other factors all argue for rapid and continuing growth.

With so convincing a scenario, it is reasonable to assume that mental health services within HMOs will grow apace. And such assumptions have come to influence the thinking about the future of mental health care in the United States. A very good case can be made. Mental health services are required of all federally qualified HMOs, the HMO is a good vehicle to bring about what health planners and policy makers have long sought—the integration of health and mental health—and mental health care within the HMO can help resolve the problems of access and stigma that have long troubled the mental health field.

All this will probably come about. Yet we think it is more than iconoclastic zeal or obsessive worry to question the conventional wisdom, to point out that, while there are strong grounds for optimism (if one assumes, as we do, that HMOs are an excellent vehicle for mental health care), all may not be so rosy. The Senate Labor and Human Resources Committee, for example, at its hearings early in 1984 refused to recommend legislation that would have required all federally qualified HMOs to provide inpatient mental health services. (Limited outpatient care has always been required.) This is not the first time, nor is it likely to be the last, that there has been something less than enthusiasm about mental health services in HMOs. There has long been resistance by some HMOs to the notion of any required mental health care. Several strong and well-organized attempts have been made to amend the HMO legislation so that all mental health care would be voluntary, a position supported (at least in the past) by the HMO trade association. So far, these efforts have not prevailed. It is still too early to tell what effect the new dominance of large for-profit companies will have on the mix of services provided by HMOs, particularly on mental health. Since several of the largest are insurance companies, their track record should not inspire a great deal of confidence.

And seasoned mental healthers have learned that we cannot rely on the public at large to help us capture the attention of either the government or the private sector about the value of mental health care in HMOs, or anywhere else for that matter. A recent experience at the Rockridge Healthplan (an HMO in the San Francisco Bay area) is a small, nondefinitive, but nagging reminder. We did a survey of several hundred employees of the University of California who had newly joined our HMO during open enrollment (the one time each year that employees can change their health coverage). Just prior to the open enrollment, we had substantially expanded the outpatient mental health coverage, and we wanted to know whether the change (the only one we made) had any influence on the decision to join. Only 7 percent said it was a major factor; 10 percent said it was somewhat a factor. The sample was small (only 182) but this is a population generally considered to be "mental health oriented," and the result tends to confirm what we already know—that public interest in and advocacy for mental health is not nearly as strong as we would like.

Perhaps this caution about the future growth of mental health services in HMOs (and in medical care generally) is too much a reflection of the past—too much the uneasy, somewhat insecure reaction of a minority accustomed to being ignored or devalued. For the experience to date of mental health services in HMOs is one of growth and progress, as we shall illustrate later on.

DEVELOPMENT

Within the past few years HMOs have become a well-recognized, if not always welcome, part of the health care scene in the United States. It took a long time. Though not designated as such, HMOs have been around in one form or another since the early 1930s, over forty years before they received formal governmental recognition through the HMO Act of 1973. In 1929 two physicians (Donald Ross and H. Clifford Loos) set up a fee-for-service group practice that primarily served employees of the city of Los Angeles. Some of these employees, concerned that they might not be able to afford the fees, persuaded Ross and Loos to take care of their families for a prepaid monthly rate of $2.00. The idea was successful and grew into an HMO that now serves over 200,000 members. The Kaiser Foundation Medical Program was started in 1933 by a surgeon who provided medical care to construction workers building an aqueduct in the southern California desert. It is now the nation's best-known HMO. Other prepaid schemes, including the Group Health Association (1937), the Health Insurance Plan of Greater New York (1947), and the Group Health Cooperative of Puget Sound (1947), helped establish prepaid health care in America (Mackie & Decker, 1981).

President Nixon's declaration in 1969 of a national "health care crisis" generated attempts to develop a solution to the problem of rising costs that would be attractive both to Democrats, who had spawned Medicare and Medicaid in 1965 and were now pushing for national health insurance legislation, and to Republicans, who were generally opposed to changes in American medicine's tradition of private enterprise. The idea of prepaid health care seemed to meet all their needs. Prepaid care would shift the financial incentives toward cost containment; the emphasis on health *maintenance* would provide further hope for cost savings; prevention had wide bipartisan appeal; and the grants under the proposed legislation would stimulate the development of HMOs in the private sector.

The HMO Act (Public Law 97-222) provided for loans and grants to organizations willing to:

1. Provide or arrange for specified inpatient and outpatient services;
2. Serve a voluntarily enrolled population;
3. Provide services for a fixed per-capita fee (paid monthly, quarterly, or annually) not related to how much services would actually be used; and
4. Assume some financial risk or gain (Luft, 1981).

The legislation required that each HMO provide a wide range of services, including office visits, hospital care, prevention, laboratory, and a maximum of twenty outpatient mental health visits. (No such limit was placed on the amount of outpatient medical visits required.) Inpatient mental health care was not included.

Many other things, including organizational structure, accessibility, membership mix, and rate setting, were included in the 1973 legislation. Any HMO that met these specifications would be designated as federally qualified and as such could qualify for loans and grants. They could also mandate any employer with twenty-five or more employees to offer the HMO as a health benefit if there was one in the area.

Although the federal support and the employer mandate were attractive, the scope of benefits required by the original legislation, as well as other restrictions, were such that few existing prepaid groups opted to become federally qualified. It was only after the 1976 amendments that HMO growth really began.

The 1973 legislation provided that HMOs be organized according to one of three models:

1. Staff type—in which all providers are employees of the HMO;

2. Group type—in which one or more groups of providers contract with the HMO (usually paid on a capitated basis) to provide services; and
3. Individual Practice Association (IPA) type—in which individual providers work in their own office and are paid by the HMO, sometimes on a fee-for-service basis.

In a later amendment a combination of these basic models was permitted.

From 1974 to 1981, $364 million in grants and loans were given to help develop HMOs. The grants paid for the costs of development—planning, construction, and so forth—and the loans for the operating losses that were almost inevitable during the first few years. In a 1978 survey, 63% (77 of the 123 HMOs responding) indicated that they had received financial assistance from the government (Levin & Glasser, 1979). In 1981, the Reagan administration stopped federal funding for HMOs, and the involvement of the private for-profit sector began to grow. Large insurance companies (e.g., Blue Cross/Blue Shield, CIGNA, Prudential) and health care companies (e.g., U.S. Health Care and Health America) entered the field. They purchased and/or affiliated with existing HMOs, a number of whom lacked the resources to grow and in some cases to survive, and they developed new HMOs. A number of hospitals established their own HMOs to help ensure a source of patients to maintain occupancy rates.

GROWTH

In 1970, when interest in federal government support for HMOs began to develop, there were 26 HMO-like prepaid systems serving just under 3 million people in the United States (Interstudy, 1983). Since then the number has climbed steadily, with the exception of a slight dip in the mid-1970s. In July 1983 there were 280 HMOs, serving 12.5 million people, about 5% of the population. California has more HMOs (32) than any other state—39% of all people who belong to HMOs live there. Wisconsin, with 19 HMOs, and Massachusetts, with 17, are next. HMO enrollment increased over 15% from June 1982 to 1983, the greatest growth since 1978. California led the nation in growth, adding over 350,000 members, followed by Massachusetts, Illinois, and Michigan. HMOs appear to be best established on the east and west coasts and least developed in the South, although much expansion is now taking place there.

Growth is expected to continue in the future, perhaps at an accelerated rate. A number of states are now encouraging or requiring Medicaid recipients and state employees to join HMOs. More and more private employers, in an effort to control what has been a rapid increase in the cost of health benefits, are promoting HMOs to their employees. And incentives may shortly give way to insistence. Just recently, the Lockheed Corporation required all new employees to join an HMO, at least for the first year of their employment.

LEGISLATIVE HISTORY

The 1973 HMO legislation, as well as the amendments in 1976, 1978, and 1981, developed in an atmosphere of political differences and controversy from which mental health services were not exempt. Originally, the House and Senate developed very different bills. The Senate committee led by Edward Kennedy drafted a comprehensive bill requiring a wide range of benefits, including social services, mental health services (to be provided in conjunction with community mental health centers whenever possible), and drug and alcohol rehabilitation. The House bill was much more modest. It specified five basic services to be required of all HMOs, as well as a long list of supplemental services that the HMO would provide only if it was paid an additional fee. Mental health and drug/alcohol addiction services were among the supplemental benefits.

Committee members in both the House and Senate were not unanimous in their support of the bills they had drafted. In the Senate committee there was concern that the required services were too broad. Congressman Hudnut, a member of the House committee, was critical of its failure to include mental health as a basic benefit. He argued that the correlation between physical health and mental health was strong and, as had been stated in the testimony of the American Psychiatric Association, by not including at least some psychiatric care in the basic benefits a disservice would be done to HMO members. He argued that, contrary to popular belief, including such services would not increase premium costs to a burdensome level and cited $7.50–$15.00 per member per year as the expected additional costs for limited psychiatric benefits.

Hudnut got what he wanted when the House and Senate versions of the bill went to conference. The House format of basic and supplemental services was retained, but the number of services was broadened to include twenty outpatient mental health visits as well as treatment and referral for alcohol and drug dependence. Psychiatric inpatient services were not mentioned. Additional mental health services were included in the supplemental list (U.S. Congress, Hearings before U.S. Senate Committee on Labor and Public Welfare and House Committee on Interstate and Foreign Commerce, 1973).

Very few HMOs in operation at the time applied for federal funds, nor did new HMOs, because they felt unable to offer the wide range of services required at a competitive price. As a result, an attempt was made to amend the legislation by deleting mental health, as well as drugs and alcohol, from the list of basic services and including only emergency and acute detoxification services. It was argued that traditional indemnity insurance plans did not cover such services. If HMOs were required to do so, they would be at a strong competitive disadvantage.

The arguments of those opposed to outpatient mental health as a basic service were not sufficiently persuasive and the amendments to the HMO Act did not change this requirement. There were further attempts by the HMO lobby to delete or at least decrease mental health benefits, but they have not been successful. The now-familiar argument that the overuse of mental health services causes them to become prohibitively expensive and uninsurable, particularly in a competitive environment, has not been true in HMOs. In fact, the great majority of nonfederally qualified HMOs provide mental health care, not because they are legally required to do so, but rather to compete with the others.

BENEFITS

Federal law mandates that any federally qualified HMO must make available to its members twenty outpatient mental health visits per year. There is no requirement for any inpatient psychiatric services. HMOs must also provide medical treatment for alcohol and drug addiction (most specifically, detoxification), as well as referral services. Since many HMOs are not federally qualified and the whole issue of mental health coverage has long been controversial, it is not surprising that there is quite a bit of variation in what is actually being provided. In a study of 205 HMOs, Levin and Glasser (1984) found that 6% of them offered no mental health benefits. Of the other 193, over 75% offered the standard twenty outpatient sessions with a mean co-payment per visit of $4.00. The co-payment was usually charged after a specified number of free visits—most commonly ten. Thirty was the median number of inpatient mental health days offered. Four percent of the HMOs offered no coverage for substance abuse, 42% covered detoxification and emergency intervention only, and the others offered more extensive services.

Utilization of mental health services by HMO members is limited by a number of mechanisms, including extra cost for supplemental mental health benefits (45%), co-payments, annual and lifetime limits, deductibles, and mandatory periods of 90 or 120 days between psychiatric admissions (Levin & Glasser, 1984).

Levin and Glasser also note that HMO age and type were significantly related to the extent of mental health benefits offered. Group and staff models, for example, offered significantly more outpatient mental health visits than IPAs. The older HMOs (11–15 years old) offered the most outpatient coverage (mean of 25.8 visits per year), and the newer ones offered less (mean of 20 visits per year for those 1–5 years old). Taken as an average, the HMOs surveyed offered a mean of 36.1 inpatient days and 21.0 outpatient visits per year. There was little difference between the federally qualified and nonqualified ones. According to Reid (1975) there is less variation in mental health services offered by HMOs than by conventional indemnity insurance plans. HMO executives report that the three most important factors influencing the extent of their mental health benefits were the desire to control inpatient psychiatric utilization and cost, compliance with state and/or federal regulations, and comparability with other HMOs in the service area.

STRUCTURE AND UTILIZATION

The HMO legislation specified the amount and kind of mental health services to be provided, but not the how. Consequently, there is a great deal of variety.

Before Levin and Glasser did their initial work in 1978, the reports on how mental health services were provided in HMOs were essentially anecdotal (Budman, 1981; Muller, 1978; Bennett, 1979; Bittker & George, 1980; Rittelmeyer & Flynn, 1978). In their later work (1984) Levin and Glasser surveyed and reported on the organizational characteristics of mental health services in HMOs.

About 19% of responding HMOs in the survey had their own internal mental health staff and 36% provided mental health services through an agreement with an outside service. Almost half (45%) stated that they had a combination of internal and external providers. In general, the larger HMOs had their own staff and the smaller ones depended on outside providers. The majority of those HMOs contracting out for mental health services depended upon private practitioners. Community mental health centers were the next most common source. Private mental health groups and clinics and university-based psychiatry departments were cited least often.

About one-third of the HMOs with their own mental health services had a separate mental health department; 27% stated that the mental health staff worked in conjunction with a health care team and/or in a liaison capacity. Larger HMOs were more likely to have separate departments than smaller ones. Not surprisingly, IPAs were least likely to utilize either of these approaches; they tended to refer their psychiatric patients to psychiatrists in private practice. While HMOs have traditionally used nonphysician mental health providers, the larger ones were most likely to do so.

Forty-five percent of the HMOs surveyed allowed their members to self-refer for mental health services, and in these, about one-third of the mental health patients were self-referred. Most of the remaining HMOs required that a primary-care physician make the referral, but indicated that virtually all such requests are approved.

The growth of HMOs has been related to their ability to provide comprehensive health care at costs considerably below those in the traditional fee-for-service practice. The major factor in these cost savings is reduced hospitalization. Hospital utilization by HMO members is far below that of subscribers to Blue Cross/Blue Shield and other indemnity plans. And it is clear that the difference results from styles of practice rather than the health status of the different patient populations (Manning et al., 1984). HMOs place greater emphasis on outpatient and preventive care and reserve hospitalization for those who cannot be cared for in any other setting (Luft, 1981).

The same appears to be true of mental health care in HMOs. In comparing prepaid practices with indemnity plans, Craig and Patterson (1981) and Reid (1975) found a shift away from inpatient toward outpatient care in the prepaid plans. In Craig and Patterson's review of published studies they found outpatient utilization to be higher in the prepaid plans. Diehr and associates (1984) did a prospective study of persons enrolling in Blue Cross, a group model HMO, and an IPA. They found, like Craig, that a higher proportion of the HMO members used the outpatient mental health service than did members of Blue Cross. But the Blue Cross members made more visits than those in the HMOs. This probably reflects the emphasis in HMOs on short-term therapy, as compared with the orientation of psychiatrists and others in private practice.

In Levin et al.'s (1984) study the mean inpatient psychiatric utilization rate was 32.1 days per 1,000 members per year, with three admissions per 1,000 members and an average length of stay of 10.2 days. Outpatient mental health visits were 0.3 per member per year. That these data are subject to wide variations is illustrated by our experience at the Rockridge Healthplan, a 25,000 member HMO with a multidisciplinary mental health department. The inpatient psychiatric utilization at Rockridge during 1983 was 9.9 days per thousand; the average length of stay, 7.8 days; and the admissions per thousand, 1.3. The outpatient mental health utilization was about the same as that in Levin's study. Given the limited amount of data available, such comparisons are speculative at best. Nonetheless, there are several things about the Rockridge program that could be contributing to our sharply lower utilization rates.

At Rockridge, the primary medical care is mostly provided by family practitioners who, by virtue of their training and personal values, are generally more sensitive to psychosocial issues than are other physicians. So they interact regularly with the mental health department, consult frequently, are alert to and work with the emotional aspects of their patients' medical problems, and recognize when their patients need the help of mental health professionals.

The mental health staff is committed to the ideology of community mental health. Rockridge members with chronic mental illness are helped to stay out of the hospital through ongoing medication maintenance clinics and groups. Medication compliance is given a great deal of attention, and the mental health staff works closely with the clinical pharmacists to help ensure that patients take their drugs properly (Meier, 1981). The Rockridge staff responds to crises very rapidly and has available a range of responses—short-term crisis-oriented psychotherapy, individual or group therapy, medication clinics, halfway houses, and inpatient care when necessary. Hospitalization is seen as a last resort, utilized only when nothing else will do. Health education classes—stress reduction, preparation for childbirth, and so forth—also contribute to the mental health program.

ADVANTAGES

The HMO seems in many ways to be very well suited for the provision of mental health services. It provides comprehensive health care in a setting where medical and mental health professionals have the opportunity to interact, consult, and co-manage patients. It has been demonstrated that there is a greater likelihood for psychiatric/emotional problems to be diagnosed when mental health and medical services are provided in the same setting (NIMH, 1983). It has also been shown that the availability of mental health services to certain subpopulations of medical patients can help reduce the inappropriate utilization of more expensive medical services (Follette & Cummings, 1967; Goldberg et al., 1970, 1981; Jones & Vischi, 1979; Mumford, Schlesinger, & Glass, 1982; White, 1981). These and other "offset studies" seem to show that mental health services are not only beneficial to patients but cost-effective as well.

The HMO environment can benefit practitioners as well as patients. Where medical and mental health staff work together there is opportunity for cross-fertilization. Physicians can develop a greater sensitivity to the psychosocial aspects of illness (Rittelmeyer & Flynn, 1978), and mental health professionals can better understand the interaction between organic and psychological components.

The HMO offers a good environment for people in need of mental health care. Because it is a general medical setting, mental health patients are less visible and therefore less concerned about stigma than they would be if seen, for example, in a psychiatric clinic. And the HMO reduces not only the psychological barriers to access, but the monetary ones as well. The mental health coverage is included in the cost—the only additional expense would be for services beyond those included in the benefit package. At a time when indemnity carriers are reducing their coverage for mental health care, this is not an insubstantial advantage.

Continuity of care is enhanced as well. It is easier for the patient's various medical and mental health providers to communicate with each other, and there is a good transfer of data because of a common medical record.

Research on such issues as the integration of health and mental health services, utilization, offset effects, treatment effectiveness, and the like is more easily done in the HMO. Because they serve a defined population that generally obtains all of its care in one setting, the problem of obtaining accurate numerators and denominators is more easily solved in HMOs. In such a setting patients can be followed fairly easily.

CONCLUSIONS

The mental health field has not always welcomed the "intrusion" of new providers (individuals or organizations) or ideologies into what it has traditionally considered to be its domain. But the growth of HMOs brings new and potentially important opportunities in research, in training, and in practice. Research questions abound and by virtue of their expertise mental health professionals are very well suited to address them. HMOs seem particularly well equipped to serve as training sites for psychologists, psychiatrists, and social workers. Such training and the linkages that develop with university departments could help enrich curricula and open up new employment possibilities. And the opportunity to practice in a comprehensive health setting, one in which prevention is both an ideology and a financial imperative, should be attractive to many mental health professionals whose values and aspirations have not been entirely fulfilled by the community mental health movement.

Whether all of this will come about is not entirely clear, but HMOs do seem to have a very promising future as providers of mental health care. We should, however, keep in mind the words of that great philosopher, Charlie Brown, who said, "There is no heavier burden than a great potential."

REFERENCES

Bennett, M. J., & Wisneski, M. J. (1979). Continuous psychotherapy within a HMO. *American Journal of Psychiatry, 136,* 1283–1287.

Bittker, T. E., & George, J. (1980). Psychiatric services options within a health maintenance organization. *Journal of Clinical Psychiatry, 41,* 192–198.

Budman, S. H. (1981). Mental health services in health maintenance organizations. In A. Broskowski et al., *Linking health and mental health.* Beverly Hills: Sage Publications.

Craig, T. J. & Patterson, D. Y. (1981). A comparison of mental health costs and utilization under three insurance models. *Medical Care, 19,* 184–192.

Diehr, P. et al. (1984). Ambulatory mental health services utilization in three provider plans. *Medical Care, 22,* 1–12.

Follette, W., & Cummings, N. A. (1967). Psychiatric services and medical utilization in a prepaid health plan setting. *Medical Care, 5,* 25–35.

Goldberg, I. D. et al. (1970). Effect of a short term psychiatric therapy benefit on the utilization of medical services in a prepaid group practice medical program. *Medical Care, 8,* 419–428.

Goldberg, I. D. et al. (1981). Utilization of medical services after short-term psychiatric therapy in a prepaid health plan setting. *Medical Care, 19,* 672–686.

Interstudy. (1983). *National HMO census: Annual report on the growth of HMOs in the U.S.* Excelsior, MN: Author.

Jones, K., & Vischi, T. R. (1979). Impact of alcohol, drug abuse and mental health treatment on medical care utilization. *Medical Care, 17* (Suppl.).

Levin, B. L., & Glasser, J. H. (1979). A survey of mental health service coverage within health maintenance organizations. *American Journal of Public Health, 69*, 1120–1125.

Levin, B. L., & Glasser, J. H. (1984). A national survey of prepaid mental health services. *Hospital and Community Psychiatry, 35*, 350–355.

Levin, B. L. et al. (1984). Changing patterns in mental health service coverage within health maintenance organizations. *American Journal of Public Health, 74*, 453–458.

Luft, H. (1981). *Health maintenance organizations: Dimensions of performance.* New York: John Wiley and Sons.

Mackie, D. L., & Decker, D. K. (1981). *Group and IPA HMOs.* Rockville, MD: Aspen.

Manning, W. G. et al. (1984). A controlled trial of the effect of a prepaid group practice on *use* of services. *New England Journal of Medicine, 310*:1505–1510.

Meier, G. (1981). HMO experiences with mental health services to the long-term emotionally disabled. *Inquiry, 18*, 125–138.

Muller, D. J. (1978). The external provision of health maintenance organization mental health services. *American Journal of Psychiatry, 135*, 735–738.

Mumford, E., Schlesinger, H. J., & Glass, G. V. (1982). The effects of psychological intervention on recovery from surgery and heart attacks: An analysis of the literature. *American Journal of Public Health, 72*, 141–151.

National Institute of Mental Health. (1983). *Use of health and mental health outpatient services in four organized health care settings.* [NIMH Series DN No. 1, DHHS Publication No. (ADM)83-859]. Rockville, MD: The Institute, 1983.

Reid, L. S. (1975). *Coverage and utilization of care for mental conditions under health insurance—Various studies, 1973–4.* Washington, DC: American Psychiatric Association.

Rittelmeyer, L. F., & Flynn, W. E. (1978). Psychiatric consultation in a HMO: A model for education in primary care. *Americal Journal of Psychiatry, 135*, 1089–1092.

U.S. Congress, House of Representatives, Committee on Interstate and Foreign Commerce, Hearings 1971–1981.

U.S. Congress, Senate, Committee on Labor and Public Welfare, Hearings 1971–1981.

White, S. L. (1981). The impact of mental health services on medical care utilization: Economic and organizational implications. *Hospital and Community Psychiatry, 32*, 311–318.

7

The New Delivery System

Nicholas A. Cummings
Leonard J. Duhl

In this brave new world of HMOs, PPOs, EPOs, IPAs, PHPs, and DRGs, only one thing is certain: the solo practice of psychotherapy as we know it today is an endangered species. Economic, social, governmental, and internal forces have all conspired to bring about its extinction, probably by the end of the decade. To be sure, relatively few psychotherapists will maintain a carriage trade and manage to hang onto what will become anachronistic practice, but most psychiatrists and psychologists will have to find alternative ways to make a living.

Fewer and fewer persons are alive today who remember the Great Depression and the stark reality that health care was hard to come by for those who could not afford it. During the last fifty years we have developed the social attitude that the best and unlimited health care is the right of all, in spite of our failure to enact a universal system of health care and our insistence that health care delivery remain vested in the private sector and under the principles of free enterprise. We have accomplished this by a pattern of third-party reimbursement to the provider by either the government or private industry, thus arriving at the same state of affairs that is found in countries that have universal, government-sponsored health care: We have all but abolished personal restraint and responsibility when we seek medical attention. At the same time medical technology has advanced to the level at which we can often sustain life almost indefinitely. Our society believes this technology should be available to all Americans, without pausing to answer the unavoidable questions of how we are going to allocate scarce resources, such as organ transplants, or who is to pay for inordinately costly procedures that can run into the hundreds of thousands of dollars per patient. These and other economic forces have escalated the inflation rate for health care at twice the rate as that for the economy as a whole. In looking for a quick and easy solution, it is easy to blame the health care provider. A restauranteur acquaintance advises, when making dinner reservations, always to put the title before your name, because everyone knows that doctors are rich and tip well. This way you will get the best table and excellent service. The part about tipping has not been borne out in our perception of our colleagues' behavior, but this vignette illustrates the extent to which the public believes doctors are rich; it should serve as a warning regarding vulnerability. An angry public seeking to cut health costs can readily scapegoat the providers.

Regarding our own fields of psychiatry and psychology, there is a growing conviction in our society that the third-party payer should reimburse not only for the treatment of emotional distress; it should also subsidize the pursuit of happiness and individual growth through unlimited psychotherapy. Adherents to this belief are not limited to patients, or, in our professions, to those practitioners associated with either psychoanalysis or the human potential movement. Without debating the merits of this belief, suffice it to say that those who must pay the bill are balking at the specter of open-ended or uncontrollable psychotherapy costs. We are clearly on the defensive.

Historically, becoming a health care provider was not the avenue toward economic privilege. The well-to-do doctor is a phenomenon of the last three or four decades, and there is every indication that the old order will return as the doctor glut increases. There are now 280 physicians for every 100,000 Americans, or twice the ratio of 1950. Compare this with the fact that there are nearly 30 psychiatrists and licensed psychologists per 100,000 Americans, or over ten times the ratio found in 1950! We have reached the saturation point without even taking into consideration the rapidly emerging mosaic of mental health care providers such as clinical social workers, psychiatric nurse practitioners, and marriage, family, and child counselors. These potential providers already exceed twice the number of psychiatrists and psychologists combined, and they are rapidly gaining statutory recognition and third-party payment privileges in state after state. The day is not far off when the word *glut* will seem insufficient to describe the horde of practitioners clamoring at the ever-shrinking market of available clients.

SOCIAL ENTREPRENEURSHIP

These forces, both external and internal to our professions, will greatly strengthen the hands of industry and government as drastic steps are taken to tether uncontrollable health costs. Cost containment will be the order of the day, and the future will rest with those who can provide services efficiently. Certainly the large health corporations will move swiftly into the market with their management skills, cost cutting, and elimination of duplication. But large corporations have one major flaw: the loss of personal care or the human touch. In the twenty-five year association of one of the authors with the Kaiser-Permanente System, he has seen growth eliminate the personal caring that the patient desires from the healer. There is no question that if one is seriously ill, he or she will receive excellent care. But gone is the important personal ingredient that seems to promote healing in the usual therapeutic encounter.

There will be room in the future for individual practitioners who would form group service delivery models that can cut costs and still maintain the quality and personal caring that are essential to the real psychological model. Unfortunately, most psychiatrists and psychologists eschew anything that smacks of business, almost as if by our very characters we gravitated to these professions. But quality care is not incompatible with efficiency, and we would submit that the psychotherapists who survive the 1980s will be the individuals who have mastered what we term "social entrepreneurship," or a melding of humanism and efficiency.

It is for those individuals, who would meet the economic and social challenge by combining personal caring with a strong business sense, thus becoming "social entrepreneurs," that this section is written.

TYPES OF DELIVERY SYSTEMS

The preferred provider organization (PPO) is a delivery model in
which a contractual arrangement has been negotiated among
payers, providers, and consumers so that health care is provided
to a defined pool of consumers at a discounted rate based on
fee-for-service. The provider benefits by receiving a steady flow
of referrals, a minimum financial risk, and regularized payments for services rendered. Mental health practitioners can
form group practices to fit a mental health PPO model, follow an
HMO model (described below), or develop an employee assistance program (EAP). As such, the group practice would contract with existing health delivery systems (indemnity carriers,
PPOs, HMOs) to provide just the mental health benefit, or arrange with large employers to provide an EAP. These practitioner groups can be nonprofit associations, or for-profit partnerships or corporations. The mental health practitioners must
be prepared to provide their services within the benefit structure of their client PPO and to accept the PPO's utilization
review and quality control systems.

The health maintenance organization (HMO) is a health care
delivery system that delivers comprehensive health care to pre-
enrolled subscribers on a prepaid basis. There are three types of
HMOs:

1. The staff model provides services through practitioners
working directly with the HMO either as employees or contractors, usually in specified central locations. In other words,
the providers do not work out of their own offices and practices.

2. In the individual practice model (IPA) providers contract
to provide specified services, usually out of their own offices. It
is usual for such providers to maintain their own part-time
private practices along with providing services to the HMO
subscribers. They can be reimbursed through fee-for-service in a
pre-arranged fee schedule, or they may be capitated.

3. In a group HMO model there is a contract, usually with
several groups of providers who agree to devote a specified
percentage of their time to the subscribers (enrollees) of the
HMO, either on a salaried or a capitated basis.

There are opportunities for mental health practitioners to
form efficient and effective group practice organizations that

will undertake the delivery of just the mental health benefit portion to the client's enrollees. Most practitioners will prefer the IPA model because it provides more autonomy than the HMO staff model. Two caveats are important, however. First, the IPA cannot effectively compete with the model with its central location, reduced costs, and constant self-monitoring. Second, as the IPA model is squeezed by the HMO or PPO, it has little alternative but to, in turn, squeeze the practitioners through lowered capitation rates or a reduced fee-for-service schedule. Nonetheless, the IPA model HMOs are presently the largest segment of the HMO industry, which in itself has been growing at an annual 15% rate.

Other considerations for practitioners interested in forming mental health HMOs or PPOs include issues of confidentiality and quality. The client organization may demand too great an access to patient information, or it may unduly subordinate quality to cost containment. Further, practitioners must be careful not to violate the professional practices acts of the various states, or to risk antitrust suits by forming closed systems of practitioners that would limit rather than enhance competition. As regards these caveats, most state medical practices acts prohibit the direct hiring of licensed providers by other than an organization owned and controlled by licensed practitioners, the practitioners must be hired as independent contractors.

Many authorities regard the PPO as a transition stage between traditional care and the efficient, effective, and more innovative HMO. They predict that within a few years the PPO-type of delivery system will disappear in favor of the HMO, which will become the model method of delivering health care.

MARKETING OR MORBIDITY

Health care has been regarded as the supreme entitlement. Americans have not wanted patients or doctors to be cost conscious and, not surprisingly, they are not (Samuelson).

All of this is changing in an environment of rising health costs and the willingness of large health corporations to introduce cost-cutting efficiency into the current nonsystem of health care delivery. These corporations, a recent phenomenon of our unstable health economy, will undoubtedly capture a significant if not major market share, but they will never succeed in staking a claim to all of health care delivery. Rapid medical technology not withstanding, Americans want their doctors to look like TV's Marcus Welby. The further the physician deviates from that image, the less the confidence on the part of the patient, no matter how much awesome apparatus surrounds the man or woman in white. Neither the corporation nor the small social entrepreneur can give America Marcus Welby, for as those of us who have watched the good doctor on TV discovered, he had only one patient per week which with to contend. But the social entrepreneur can still dispense a lot more TLC and downright human concern than can the corporation. This is your greatest selling point, if at the same time you can offer a cost/therapeutically effective treatment package.

Even the best program will fail without proper marketing. The key to social entrepreneurship will be marketing, and "marketing or morbidity" will be the practitioner's version of the academician's slogan, "publish or perish." It will be strictly a buyer's market, with the practitioner having to demonstrate that better mental health care can be delivered more efficiently and at less cost.

Psychologists and psychiatrists must learn to market themselves if they are to succeed, and market research is essential to a successful marketing program. You just have to be sure that what you think you are selling is what other people think they are buying. Only fools and a lot of well-meaning practitioners would delude themselves into believing they could define their goals, identify the consumer's need, and target a package without the help of a marketing expert. This expertise is readily available and is as important early on as is the attorney who draws up your business agreements for you, your fellow participants, and your clientele.

TAILORING YOUR PACKAGE OF BENEFITS

After years of rising health costs, hospitals have finally been pushed off the dole and into competition. This will soon happen to practitioners, and the process will cause considerable pain. Many will not survive the shock.

Psychologists and psychiatrists must stop thinking of third-party reimbursement as a cornucopia by which anything goes and everything will be reimbursed because, after all, the practitioner knows best what the patient needs. If research tomorrow were to demonstrate that psychoanalysis is the most effective treatment for all patients with emotional problems, it still could not be marketed because of its inordinate cost.

What, then, can the practitioner realistically offer? His cues come from Malan (1963, 1976), Cummings (1977), and Cummings and VandenBos (1979). Malen, working in Great Britain under socialized medicine, discovered that brief therapy works with therapists who believe in brief therapy. Cummings, working for a quarter of a century at Kaiser-Permanente in San Francisco, found that therapists who believe in brief therapy are those who are trained in the techniques of brief therapy, regardless of their original orientation and previous adherence to long-term practice. In fact, in reporting eighteen years of research, Cummings further found that when a workable brief therapy model is offered, and without any prior screening for suitability, 85% of the patients will select brief therapy and will improve significantly with short-term treatment. Only 10% will self-select long-term therapy and most will need that more protracted intervention. The implication is obvious: with 85% of patients profiting from brief therapy, the 10% who require longer-term treatment should receive it if this can be financed.

With most practitioners a much larger proportion of their patients are in long-term therapy. It may very well be that this is iatrogenic rather than natural. One of the present authors recalls that, years ago, his skills as a psychotherapist had developed to such a point that, with an appropriate interpretation or intervention, he could prevent any patient who was considering terminating from doing so. There followed a painful period of soul-searching: Was this skill being utilized for the benefit of the patient or the practitioner?

There remain the 5% of the total therapy population, reported by Cummings in his eighteen years of research, who proved to be interminable. This is the psychotherapy group that terrifies every third-party payer and provides a virtual annuity for some psychologists and psychiatrists. Every provider must develop effective techniques for dealing with the interminable patient. Otherwise, the mental health package will not be cost-effective.

Most third-party payers use artificial means to limit abuse. These artificial means, as contrasted with therapeutic strate-

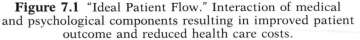

Figure 7.1 "Ideal Patient Flow." Interaction of medical and psychological components resulting in improved patient outcome and reduced health care costs.

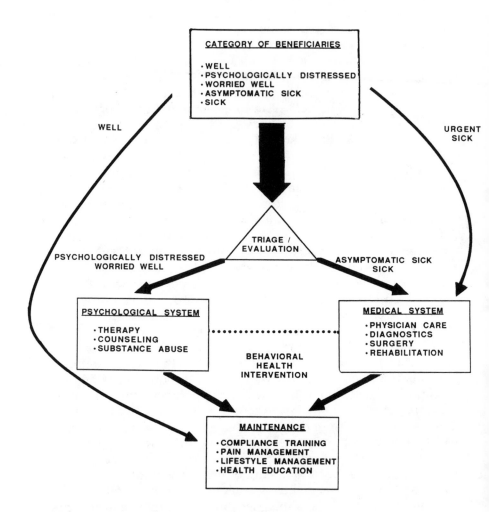

gems, include first-dollar amounts, limitations on number of sessions, or co-insurance where the patient pays one-half or more of the fee. We are opposed to these approaches because they often jettison the treatment before it has been accomplished. We do favor brief therapy skills that effectively and efficiently do the job and result in patient satisfaction.

Most psychiatrists and psychologists practicing today will require retraining in the newer brief therapies before they can become competitive. It has long been the misfortune of the psychotherapy professions that the patient receives whatever the therapist is trained to render (psychoanalysis, behavior modification, etc.) regardless of the patient's presenting condition. The maturity of any profession is measured by the number of specifics it has available. Medicine came of age with the discovery of a wide repertoire of specifics; thus antibiotics are specifics for pneumonia, and so forth. Most practitioners provide one form of treatment modality for all their patients and are unaware that psychology and psychiatry have developed a wider range of specific treatments. These specifics are the models that meld dynamic therapy, behavioral technique, and systems approaches into targeted brief therapies.

DESIGNING YOUR DELIVERY ORGANIZATION AND MODEL

It is apparent from the foregoing that a competitive provider will be a group practice. This does not mean the traditional group practice, which consists of a number of independent practitioners practicing under one roof and sharing expenses. Rather, it means a multimodal group practice of practitioners who can pool a broad array of therapeutic skills into an efficient organizational delivery system that contracts with third-party payers to be their preferred provider organization (PPO). These can be either carefully designed partnerships or corporations, the advantage of the latter being that liability, except for malpractice, is limited to the assets of the corporation. They can be designed toward the independent practice association (IPA) model or toward the health maintenance organization (HMO) model.

Most psychiatrists and psychologists will prefer the IPA because it gives the illusion that one retains his or her freedom. Under this model practitioners continue to practice out of their own offices and contract with other such practitioners to treat the patients of the IPA and in the manner specified in the agreement. One advantage of this model is the greater personal freedom accorded the practitioner. Another advantage is that it

is applicable to rural settings where there is not enough of a
population concentration to warrant the creation of a center, or
where the number of enrollees is thin and widely spaced geographically. By contracting with practitioners who are in their
own widely scattered offices, the thinly dispersed beneficiaries
can be serviced geographically.

The disadvantage of the IPA is its vulnerability to failure because of the difficulty of maintaining quality control over widely scattered practitioners holding on to their little turfs, and
the fact that the model is generally not as cost-effective as
the HMO and thus not as competitive. In urban and especially in
metropolitan areas the IPA will not compete favorably with the
mental health HMO (MHHMO) that can construct well-staffed
centers in strategic locations. The MHHMO model provides the
ultimate in quality control and efficiency because all practitioners are practicing together in one center under a center
director who maintains quality control through regular case
conferences.

An exclusive provider organization (EPO) is a PPO that has
negotiated an agreement wherein the eligibles must take all of
their mental health delivery from that PPO. Under a preferred
rather than exclusive status, the enrollees have a choice of two
or more PPOs or delivery systems with which the third-party
payer has contracted.

Both of these models, and variations thereof, give the emer-
gent social entrepreneur ownership and profit sharing as alternatives to future survival by becoming a practitioner for
a large health corporation. As competition heats up, it is our
prediction that many practitioners will join these corporations.
Others will form PPOs, only to fail as one of the many casualties
that are bound to dot the professional landscape as our society
moves away from solo practice to the new delivery system. One
interesting alternative involves becoming part of a national
delivery system that enables the local provider to remain small
and retain individual caring and concern for the patient.

THE SOCIAL HMO

The social health maintenance organization (HMO) would ex-
tend the concept of the HMO to include a range of social

services, such as shut-in services for the elderly. These have attracted considerable interest among psychiatrists and psychologists, as well as social scientists generally. A number of demonstration projects had been underway. However, in the summer of 1984 the Reagan administration, seeking to contain health costs and fearing a drastic increase in Medicaid and Medicare costs brought on by the acceptance of such a far-reaching concept, put the brakes on the SHMO demonstrations. For the immediate future it would appear that such demonstration projects that do continue will be funded by private foundations. At this point, the immediate future of the SHMO is not clear, and it may be that for the time being government and industry are prepared to pay only for a strict and limited definition of health care. The SHMO may be an idea whose time has not yet come.

AN ILLUSTRATIVE EXAMPLE

For purposes of illustration, the authors have adapted the organizational model from an existing statewide health delivery system located in the Midwest. The relationship is schematically presented in Figure 7.2.

The parent organization is a traditional indemnity carrier that has been in existence for three decades. Recently this carrier changed from a not-for-profit organization to a for-profit corporation, and shortly thereafter created its own HMO for a substantial portion of its business. This HMO is a wholly owned subsidiary of the parent corporation, which moved itself into the new delivery system in this manner. The HMO, in turn, contracts with the parent organization for its marketing, billing, actuarial, financial, and membership services.

For the actual delivery of the benefits to its enrollees, the HMO contracts with several medical groups, which are either partnerships of physicians or service corporations owned by participating physicians. These groups are capitated at a rate that represents 85% of usual and customary costs according to an agreed-upon fee schedule. The HMO also contracts with its participating hospitals for its inpatient care, and the medical group share in 50% of the "upside risk" for hospitalization. The total of the medical groups' risks is capped at 110%. Thus, if the

Figure 7.2 An illustration of the relationship of a mental
health maintenance organization (MHMO) to the overall
delivery of health services in a new delivery system
(adapted from an actual statewide organizational structure).

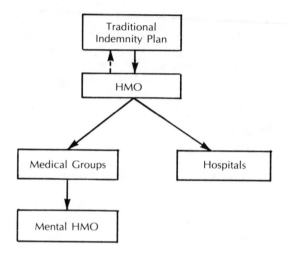

loss to the medical groups reaches this figure, the contract is
renegotiated. In this manner the medical groups are protected
from catastrophic business loss, but the incentive is toward
efficiency and away from unnecessary services, especially unnecessary hospitalization.

The medical groups provide all of the medical outpatient
services and emergency room care, but do not provide their own
psychiatric and psychological direct intervention. This is provided through a contract with a mental health maintenance
organization (MHMO), which specializes in focused, targeted
psychological interventions but also provides comprehensive
mental health services, including substance abuse programs,
and long-term therapy for those conditions which require it.
Also provided by the MHMO is an outreach program that addresses high health utilization by somaticizers and triages the

"worried well" out of the health system. The MHMO is also at risk for the psychiatric hospitalization.

A brief description of the MHMO would be useful. This particular MHMO is a part of a national for-profit MHMO with similar contracts in other states. The practitioners are licensed psychologists and board-certified psychiatrists who work in a staff model, but as independent contractors. Each center in the staff model has six to eight practitioners serving 40,000 to 60,000 enrollees of the HMO. The MHMO is capitated and receives no fee-for-service whatsoever. All providers receive 130 hours of intensive training initially, and one full year of in-service training thereafter. The centers and the practitioners are highly monitored throughout their services by clinical case conferences and computer tracking. The practitioners are eligible for profit sharing beyond the liberal base compensation. By employing focused, strategic, and targeted interventions developed in over more than twenty-five years of empirical research, the MHMO is able to offer efficient, comprehensive services with no additional cost to the patient and no limitations on the number of sessions or services.

SUMMARY

Social and economic forces, as well as factors within the professions of psychiatry and psychology, are combining to render solo practice as we now know it extinct within this decade. Cost containment will be the order of the day as our society seeks drastic measures to bring an out-of-control health economy under one leash. Large health corporations will capture a significant market share of the health industry, but there will still be room for the psychologist and psychiatrist who can learn social entrepreneurship and add to cost-effectiveness the desired human caring that a large corporation cannot provide. To form PPOs, either of the IPA or HMO models, legal, marketing, and organizational expertise will be required. There are also national organizations that will be organizing groups of practitioners into local PPOs that can retain much of the smallness and identity desired by most practitioners and patients. These local PPOs will be able to compete favorably with the large corporations only if a wide range of targeted programs, or specifics, is employed within broad, brief therapy skills. There will be interesting challenges and important opportunities for the social entrepreneur, but unfortunately there will be many failures that could have been prevented with optimal use of expertise.

REFERENCES

Cummings, N. A. (1977). The anatomy of psychotherapy under national health insurance. *American Psychologist, 32*(9): 711–718.

Cummings, N. A. (1986). The dismantling of our health system: Strategies for the survival of psychological practice. *American Psychologist, 41*(4): 426–431.

Cummings, N. A., & VandenBos, G. R. (1979). The general practice of psychology. *Professional Psychology, 10*(4): 430–440.

Malan, D. H. (1963). *A study of brief psychotherapy.* New York: Plenum Press.

Malan, D. H. (1976). *The frontier of brief psychotherapy.* New York: Plenum Press.

Samuelson, R. J. (1984, May 14). *Newsweek.*

8

Who Can Do Therapy?

Luther P. Christman

WHO CAN DO THERAPY?

The question might be better rephrased as, "Who needs therapy?" In a heterogeneous society such as the United States, the range of subtleties of behavior is so wide as to be practically unmeasurable. Furthermore, the complexities of the societal issues that persons must cope with will increase markedly as the nation moves from a post-industrial to a knowledge society. Everyone will be dealing more and more with conceptual entities at levels of abstraction often elusive of easy management. It is predictable that tension, uneasiness, and inability to manage real-life phenomena effectively will grow in incidence, even though people are better educated and have high-technology mechanisms to provide more complete information on which to base decisions. The requirements of therapy must be shaped and organized according to this scenario for the near future.

The stratification of society into many socioeconomic classes will not be a handicap to good therapy if numerous other variables can be managed better. Race, gender, religious beliefs, political orientations, life-style patterns, ethnic moorings, job mobility opportunities, and similar societal variables tend to constrict allowable behaviors and dictate what are considered as "sane" behaviors. The stressors may produce an infinity of nuances. As a result, the limitations these variables place on degrees of freedom of personal expression will contribute to the building of inter- and intrapersonal strain. The interplay of the configuration of societal norms held by the patient with those held by the therapist is an equation that predicts the degree of ease or difficulty in forming therapeutic alliances. A crucial element in establishing rapport between both persons in this dyad is the social fit of the therapy in which they are engaged. The congruency factor emanating from the selective perceptions of both will tend to bear heavily on the course of the therapeutic process. The greater the congruency, the higher the ease of facilitation of each other's efforts toward the common goal of ultimate resolution of the patient's problems. Therapeutic alliances with patients are ephemeral as well as problematic unless a high degree of agreement occurs on the entire set of variables around therapy, rather than just a consensus on techniques and professional identity.

The demand system of patients, deriving from social constrictions, is a major key to the type of therapist best suited to each. Psychotherapy, when analyzed rigorously by the canons of science, is far from an exact science. Although psychotherapy stems from scientific roots in the various behavioral sciences, differences in choices of therapeutic strategies and the accompanying styles of implementation have their origin in each therapist's knowledge system and personal history. The therapist's predisposition to ways of acting in the clinical situation is tied strongly to the nature of basic preparation. Because every therapist can use only the knowledge she/he possesses, there are stricter limitations on potential competence than are usually acknowledged. Art, therefore, becomes a prime consideration in effectively managing every therapeutic endeavor. Furthermore, the role overlap of knowledge among professions may be greater than generally conceded. These conditions, coupled with the fact that a wider range of competence probably exists within each professional group as well as among professions, produce an interesting variable. When competence is viewed in this manner, patients are provided with a larger available number of therapists than otherwise might be recognized. The wider the range of effective options, the more likely patients will be able to select therapists who meet their needs.

These distinctions, however, are not readily accepted by persons doing therapy because of staked and guarded boundaries. One observer comments:

> It is a truism that persons view the world of work through selective perceptions brought about by the kind of training they have undergone. Since all have been socialized into the role of their own discipline by a process that tends to develop strong professional biases, they have a predisposition to see the problem and their respective roles in it with decided differences. Subtle distinctions in the definition of the situation and the programs of care are almost certain to occur (1).

Comparisons of therapeutic abilities are judged using this structured thought pattern, with reality for each practitioner defined in such a manner.

The role expression of knowledge often gives heightened coloration to the perception of who is qualified to do therapy. Even though scientific theory and content do not change their characteristics and nature, the role expression of that scientific knowledge creates stylistic differences that may artificially exaggerate the perception of competency levels among different types of practitioners. The legalisms that describe and practically mandate differences in the role construction of each category of therapists reinforce stereotypical conclusions about the efficacy of respective types. Training in scientific theory and content, moreover, becomes a free marketplace open to all comers aspiring to avail themselves of equal amounts in whatever desirable mix. Additionally, the imaginative use of that knowledge cannot be easily transmitted by training. Thus, the art of practice varies highly with the ability to be imaginative and innovative, unrestricted to any one discipline or profession. Even with those of similar educational background, a Bell curve of knowledge expression begins to appear around discrete differences in the user's ability to be creative in applying knowledge in the clinical situation. Thus, the stage is set for developing decided differences in clinical competence within and among members of professions. Beutler states that:

> Effective therapists might be distinguished from ineffective ther-
> apists, not by their skill in the use of one or another technique, but
> in the timing, integration, and patterning of these strategies (2).

Because imaginative abilities always appear to be in short supply, no one profession can claim a large corner of this market. A
rich background in behavioral and biological sciences is basic to
understanding the problems presented by patients.

The growth of clinical competence in the professions has not
occurred at a uniform rate. Physicians set the pace originally,
but increasing numbers from other professions are pursuing
educational pathways leading to clinical expertise. Thus, physicians who are not psychiatrists, especially those regularly involved in primary care, as well as the more thoroughly trained
psychiatrists are the most traditionally acknowledged therapists. It appears that this role will be enhanced with the steady
increase in and use of drugs that specifically affect the neuro-
biochemistry of the central nervous system. The intense, in-
depth training in a wide range of behavioral theories has given
credence to clinical psychologists. This observation is supported
by a prodigious amount of research in this field. A similar
development is the emergence of clinical doctorates in the nursing profession, producing a small critical mass of therapists who
understand the biological and behavioral aspects of patient
symptoms as well as the pharmacological therapy employed to
modify behavior. The number of nurses prepared in this fashion
will continue to grow and will increase the population of therapists available to potential patients. Social workers and pastor-
al counselors trained at the doctoral level are also on the increase. In all likelihood, sociologists and anthropologists may
become candidates to join the ranks of psychotherapists if the
present trend of developing some members as applied scientists
continues. Members of both groups have strong behavioral science content. The trend will depend on whether those interested
in being applied scientists will combine it with clinical training.
Abilities to assess patients will be uneven and will depend, to a
large extent, on the total amount of fundamental science each
type inculcates into its training design.

It would be naive to attempt an all-inclusive list. One can
be suggestive only because the demand of the large number of

persons seeking counseling, brief therapy, and intensive and extensive care is greater than any one profession can meet. An additional variable in this equation is the degree to which organizations have increasingly sought to make the choice of who will do therapy. Over a long period of time, state legislatures have enacted licensure laws that regulate the practice of therapy. More recently, organizations such as health maintenance organizations (HMOs) find themselves in the business of providing therapeutic services. As businesses, they are concerned not only with meeting the basic requirements of licensing laws (and federal certification), but in being cost-effective as well. As a result, HMOs nationally are using an innovative mix of professional persons to provide mental health services (3). In an economic and competitive society, it can be expected that the usual marketplace phenomena will be at play. All the mechanisms are in place to stimulate the growth of types rather than to curtail entry into the field. In addition, software programs are available to the public for home computer use that will stimulate more self-help. One clinician has suggested the use of a total cybernetic diagnostic system on an epic scale (4). For the generation growing up in the computer culture, the concept of computer-assisted therapy may have appeal.

Perhaps an acceptable resolution of the social right to function as a therapist will be reached when psychotherapy becomes more scientific. Far from realization at this stage is the scientific codification of psychotherapeutic knowledge into theoretical constructs that predict outcomes with an accuracy similar in strength and exactness to those employed in the physical sciences. Hence, the precision of measurement and the methods of prescribed training required to master the subject are lacking. This gap in scientific certitude fosters the use of private opinion over the rigorous employment of science. It is difficult to exclude entrants into the field when selective perceptions and art abound more than science. Schon asserts:

> The dilemma of rigor or relevance may be dissolved if we can develop an epistemology of practice which places technical problem solving within a broader context of reflective inquiry, shows how reflection-in-action may be rigorous in its own right, and links that art of practice in uncertainty and uniqueness to the scientists' art of research (5).

Until this large scientific void is adequately filled, the range of types of practitioners claiming the right to fill it probably will be on the increase. Thus, the discipline(s) that is (are) able to lay claim to making psychotherapy more scientific, may also lay claim to being the "true practitioner(s)."

The inability so far to prove the scientific legitimacy of psychotherapy, such current issues as deregulation and the opening up of competition, and the growth in alternative forms of health care are creating a milieu that will be more consumer driven than provider controlled. Additional issues include the consumer movement, feminist movement, affirmative action proceedings, emerging equality-of-work motifs, the effect of the mass media on opinion formation, and growing skepticism about professional omnipotence in the affairs of man. In this setting, the proliferation of choices of desired care and appropriate providers will not easily lead to curtailment of types. Instead, the various professions that fit into the many different "market" niches will have some leverage in filling the wide range of therapeutic demands. The basic requirement of those who believe they are therapists will be to establish a strong scientific and clinical base for their practice, in concert with deftness in timing, integrating, and patterning of the therapeutic process in order to gain the credibility of the public that is served.

REFERENCES

1. Christman, L. (1969). Community Resources—The role of other professionals. *MCV Quarterly 5*(3), 145.
2. Beutler, L. B. (1983). Eclectic psychotherapy. New York: Pergamon Press, p. 7.
3. Chiefetz, D. I. & Salloway, J. C. (1984). Patterns of mental health services provided by HMOs. *American Psychologist, 39*(5), 495.
4. Lesse, S., (1983). A cybernated health-science diagnostic system—An urgent imperative. *American Journal of Psychotherapy, 27*(40), 451–455.
5. Schon, D. A. (1983). *The reflective practitioner.* New York: Basic Books, p. 69.

9

The Ethics of
Mental Health Practice

Anne Hartwig
Burr Eichelman

This chapter addresses ethical issues in the distribution and character of mental health care raised by the increase in health care plans such as health maintenance organizations (HMOs). While many ethical issues encompass psychiatric practice, we feel that the most significant ones can be seen in the context of economic terms and discussed ethically in terms of the just distribution of resources. This chapter is written as if mental health resources are finite, essentially limited as they are at present, with distribution requiring allocations that do not meet all expressed needs. This perspective is based on current political realities; we choose not to debate the morality of a federal budget that has increased allocations for research on national defense for 1984 by a figure that is approximately 39% of the entire estimated federal outlay for health in 1983 (1, 2). Social allocations need not be fixed at present levels, but a substantial change toward a less militaristic and more humanitarian environment is needed; but as this does not appear imminent, we shall proceed with the given of "finite" resources.

A GENERAL RIGHT TO HEALTH CARE

Medical ethicists have been at odds for some time over the issue of whether health care is an intrinsic right. Perhaps this debate has best been summarized in the report of the President's Commission for the Study of Ethical Problems in Medical and Biomedical and Behavioral Research (3).

That commission carefully avoided an assertion of health care as a right, in part because such claims are often (mis-) understood as open ended. However, the commission did argue that advanced societies—in particular, their governments—have an obligation to act as guarantors of last resort for at least the rudiments of decent health care. The extent of this obligation depends upon a host of factors, including the state of the economy, but the commitment to decent care stands as an ethical baseline.

The commission's recommendation, then, was deliberately imprecise; and its report papered over substantial differences of opinion among the philosophers and health planners whose views it invited. Still, a consensus favoring a central regulation seems to exist in this country, and we must work from this point in considering the ethics of the distribution of mental health care.

There are several popularly expressed ethical positions regarding just distribution of resources encompassed within the philosophical rubric of distributive justice. The utilitarian position of Mill (4) allocates resources to provide the greatest possible balance of good over evil, but leaves us debating whether a great deal of "good" for one is of greater or lesser worth than a bit of good for many. Marx proposed a distribution to each according to his or her need. Here the debate can begin as to the allocation of resources to the "infinitely needy" versus those who only need a band-aid to remain functional and return to health. Rawls (5) has expressed the position that an ethical distribution of resources works to the benefit of the disadvantaged.

APPLYING AN ETHICAL "CALCULUS"—SPECIAL ISSUES IN PSYCHIATRY

Even if philosophers and health planners could decide on the just means of dividing resources, mental health treatment still has special issues. The first of these is effectiveness. Treatment of pneumococcal pneumonia can be evaluated by the clearing of the lung field, a lysis of the fever, and drop in respiratory rate. Successful treatment of congestive heart failure can be assessed by a decrease in cardiomegaly and hepatomegaly and the loss of pedal edema. Treatment of mental disorders is less clearly defined, and the endpoint of treatment often is not obvious. Frequently there is not more than the patient's subjective report to evaluate changes in hallucinations, dysphoria, or anxiety. Which is the more successful treatment: removing the auditory hallucinations of a schizophrenic patient who is still too autistic to work, or returning such a patient to employment in spite of troublesome hallucinations? When has the "divorcing" patient learned enough about him- or herself in this situational disturbance to avoid recapitulating the same scenario in a new relationship? Since dynamic psychotherapy is so difficult to evaluate, should it be more or less financed in comparison with the pharmacologic or behavioral interventions in which endpoints and success or failure can be more quantitatively assessed?

More likely than not, the application of any sort of distributive calculus will require increasing evidence of tangible (measurable) success. Thus we envision a shifting of mental health treatment goals, even if ethically allocated, away from intangibles such as happiness, understanding, or contentment, toward more externally observable criteria such as return to work, maintenance of normal sleep, and return to acceptable modes of relating. Quality-of-life issues and misunderstanding of motivations may well be overlooked and unfunded because they cannot be measured and the efficacy of treatment to affect these issues cannot be assessed.

This leads us to the related issue of whether mental health problems are health (medical) problems at all. The application of the term *medical*, which grew "fat" in the days of unquestioned reimbursement, is bound to be forced onto a crash diet. People expecting to be received with open arms by psychiatrists will be told that they simply are not sick. Problems in living and their understanding may indeed by considered "psychological," that is, related to the study and understanding of the psyche, but they may come to be considered an educational, not a health, problem. Thus, the health maintenance organization (HMO) provider may accept the treatment of a manic episode with lithium as a medical problem, while refusing to accept as medical the problem of a woman who wants to understand more about her relationship with men in order to avoid entering into maladaptive relationships with them. A therapy concern can suddenly become a debatable issue when an HMO contracts to provide prepaid psychiatric (translated "medical") care for a client; whether the discovery that many psychological problems will not be treated under HMOs will affect the development and widespread adoption of HMOs remains to be seen. For example, do HMO subscribers know that the financial "break even" point for many HMOs in psychiatry is significantly less than the twelve sessions of "brief psychotherapy" described by such therapists as Sifneos (6)?

Psychiatry is also being affected by the wave of for-profit hospitals. The degree to which the population of these hospitals will be controlled by third-party authorizations or the patient's ability to pay remains to be determined, but psychiatry, with its elastic definitions of medical need, is an area in which the pursuit of well-insured or well-healed patients is less likely to be held in check by cost–benefit calculations.

Moreover, payment schedules are becoming diagnosis related, as illustrated by the movement toward diagnostically related groups (DRGs). In the inpatient DRG system, psychosis yields higher reimbursement and has more lenient trim points than do borderline personality disorders (7). Will this encourage overdiagnosing of psychotic disorders, with the potential of stigmatizing patients? How will the patient be treated who has exceeded the normative period for hospitalization such that the hospital starts to lose money? Both advocates and critics of the DRG system agree that economic motivations have become more important determinants of treatment than they previously had been. The ethical issue inherent in this development is whether such economic determination of treatment by funding produces a just distribution of resources. It arguably produces a superficially equal standardized distribution but whether it is equitable—i.e., (1) produces the most good (Mill), (2) provides the most to the most needy (Marx), or (3) assists the most disenfranchised population (Rawls)—remains to be observed. Merely linking treatment more tightly to financial issues does not in and of itself provide an unethical system in relation to the distribution of resources. However, in a for-profit hospital—

which may view a psychiatrist as an investment, given the general system of reimbursement—there seems to be potential for a conflict of interest for the therapist dealing with a sick patient whose hospitalization exceeds the DRG trim point or the HMO break-even point. The physician who has too many patients over the DRG trim point risks being replaced by a doctor whose practice more closely matches the fiscal demands of the hospital. Clinicians might then admit less disturbed psychotic patients and also less situationally disturbed patients with low funding priority. Potential consequences of this could be (1) decreased service to the situationally disturbed who only need a "band-aid" or brief hospitalization to begin coping again and (2) decreased service to the severely ill nonresponding psychotic patient. In the first example, the utilitarian ethic would be endangered; in the second example, both Marxian and Rawlsian justice are disregarded.

Time-limited HMOs and DRG programs work best financially if the noninsistent or reluctant patient is ignored. The dynamic psychotherapist who after several sessions enters into a heated transference neurosis with his or her patient and finds this patient canceling the next appointment is faced with a conflict. Should the therapist actively persuade the patient to "work through" the transference, which requires many more expensive sessions and may cause the HMO to lose money, or terminate therapy, with the patient knowing that it was incomplete but thereby allowing the HMO to make money?

There is little incentive in the future systems of time-limited therapy for a therapist to pursue the painfully slow treatment of a chronic schizophrenic who may be ambivalent about therapy and social contacts. These patients seem destined to be dropped from private health care plans and become an increasing financial demand on the public sector. As part of the public sector, they will become the patients of the community mental health systems, which are becoming more inadequately staffed and more burdened. State and county funding for psychiatric consultation by private practitioners pays approximately half of the private community hourly rate for psychiatric services (8). Moreover, there is no assurance that these agencies would be blocked from contracting for HMO services for their payees, which might further limit care for the severely mentally ill. One is struck by the potential parallel with visit-limited psychotherapy and HMOs closed to the unemployed that followed the rapid deinstitutionalization and closing of state hospitals; the result was the release of many dependent and disabled patients into communities ill prepared for them, fostering the generation of board and care homes that would lock their tenants out during the daytime to roam the streets until evening (9).

WHAT IS THE ETHICAL PROGNOSIS?

We believe that the ethical prognosis is grim. The resources made available for care may result in an increasing control of treatment predicated upon fiscal expediency rather than clinical judgment, with the result of diminished care for the neediest and potentially increased availability of care for those with more ample resources. To be sure, there is nothing new or unique about an excess of need over resources. Inequities existing at a time of relative plenty, however, can be explained away as problems not quite yet resolved and as projects of the future. When reduction rather than growth lies ahead, these hopes are not available and the unfairness is patent.

Even more disturbing are the actual patterns of triage that emerge in a system like our own. While the philosophers have yet to provide us with a fully satisfactory theory of the just distribution of mental health resources, we know something is suspect if the first group to be abandoned is the severely mentally ill, as seen with the challenges to Social Security disability benefits.

What trends will emerge given the changes in the delivery of health care? There seems little likelihood that the trend toward HMOs and DRGs will be reversed without a thorough social trial. As a consequence, we fear that once again our society will begin to develop a population of patients whom nobody wants to treat, who are too disenfranchised to complain, and whose quality of life will be demeaning and dehumanizing, perhaps with the added risk of being added to the criminal justice system. Another consequence might be development of a mental health treatment establishment that would provide inadequate treatment, not subject to monitoring of care (i.e., quality control), to those least able to complain about the treatment received. Since we believe that the mental health dollar will continue to shrink relative to the GNP and to the total health dollar, we expect the following changes in statistics: increases in (1) suicide, (2) convictions for petty crime, (3) the number of street people, and (4) substance abuse as patients seek to medicate themselves.

RESPONSES TO INEQUITIES

A system of checks and balances for monitoring of health care delivery has not, for the most part, been included in the initial phases of allocation of resources. Traditionally health care providers have utilized physicians and others involved in direct care, as well as financial advisers, to assist in the determination of expenditures and reimbursement rates for specific treatments. Legal advice might also have been sought to ensure that administrative procedures and regulations were properly included in any proposed HMO health care plan. The more recent trend has been to rely heavily upon statistical data that reports use by recipients, perhaps by diagnostic category (7), and to use this data to predict anticipated usage; obviously, fiscal analysis is a crucial component of any allocation of resources. However, a system that analyzes the tangible, quantifiable data for allocation determination but also contrasts them to the often intangible elements of ethical consequences is lacking. Probability theory does not take into account the individual. As a consequence, there is no provision for the ethical treatment of the individual exceptional case.

The existing protections or safeguards that are available to redress unethical distribution of health care resources are those that address the process by which health care is provided. Frequently these are neither known nor widely publicized to the public. A consumer or recipient of a health care plan may not know that there exists a mechanism that allows him or her to protest. The users have a right to address the board of directors of an HMO, for example, and to complain that the amount of dollars or visits allowed for a given psychiatric treatment are inadequate. The anticipated administrative response would be for the board to establish a committee to investigate the complaint, compare its findings with the complainant's charges, and propose a solution that might or might not result in either more dollars or extended visits. The reality is that this mechanism is rarely used; moreover, it is often the case that the most severely mentally ill are those most adversely affected by improper allocations and least able to use the cumbersome complaint process.

The more popular way of complaining is to do so to the therapist. Most consumers or patients would view this as an appropriate way of voicing their dissatisfaction, expecting that the therapist might be able to modify either the diagnosis or treatment plan so that the patient's needs could be met. Certainly, if the patient/consumer felt that harmful treatment had been given or that there had been negligence in the care received, the consumer could bring a malpractice action against the individual therapist and/or hospital or clinic. This option is found in the body of law known as torts, which provides a number of legal theories, such as negligence, to redress harms. Whether a patient could also cite the HMO for failure to provide sufficient resources so as to have prevented the harm initially is unclear and too speculative to discuss here.

A group of consumers who felt that they were misled by incomplete or misleading advertisements regarding their HMO provisions could use the traditional means of legal redress by bringing a civil action alleging false advertisement. Such an example might be an advertisement that claimed user access to named therapists who, in reality, were not or might never be available to the consumer. Agencies that are available for consumer protection might also be involved in administrative complaints that an entire clinic or hospital is mishandling its HMO contract. Legal and other recourses might be available if there were additional factors involving receipt of federal funds, mishandling of consumer dollars, or mismanagement or poor administration involving an HMO plan.

The reader quickly sees the problems inherent in the so-called safeguards and protections afforded the patient/consumer. First, there is the obvious observation that something must go wrong that results in harm or potential harm to someone. Second, all of the protection mechanisms require the ability to organize a complaint, knowledge of to whom the complaint should be directed, and perseverance until some resolution is reached. Third, the procedures are cumbersome and time consuming. The extraordinary amount of time involved in any administrative complaint is enough to deter all but the most persistent of consumers. The question of who funds the cost of a grievance or complaint remains unsettled. Is the cost to be borne by the individual, which might seem to be unduly harsh and predictably could lead to fewer complaints, or is it to be added to the cost of the HMO and distributed to all the consumers? The legal avenue of using the judiciary or courts to provide relief seems to be the least effective safeguard, given overburdened court calendars, high legal costs (including attorneys' fees), and lack of expertise that a court is likely to have regarding allocation of treatment plans or therapy. One must also be aware that although a court might recommend certain changes or modifications, there is no monitoring mechanism readily available to ensure that the court's plan will be followed.

There exists a parallel system of safeguards and protection for the therapist and those involved in direct patient care. The therapists initially can, through negotiation with an HMO, try to obtain more latitude by reserving some discretion in the establishment of care plans to allow for either more funds or more time for the patient. Therapists can address the board of directors or managers of the HMO by formal presentations explaining the nature of their complaints, particularly if no latitude or discretion was given to them. If, after some use of the HMO, the therapists have had complaints from their patients, these comments can be presented to the HMO directorship. If dissatisfied with an HMO, physicians and others can form an HMO of their own and attempt to market it and make it available to the consumer pool.

There is also the option for the therapist to advise the patient about the shortcomings of the HMO plan as it relates to the patient's care or treatment. Whereas in an area of medical practice such as surgery this might seem to be a viable option, one must question the advisability of discussing, in the initial contacts with a patient suffering from manic-depressive illness, the therapist's perceived need for therapy to continue beyond a twenty-visit ceiling provided through an HMO. Moreover, for example, in Madison, Wisconsin, therapists are negotiating in advance with patients, taking them into treatment only if they agree to supplement their HMO plans upon the plan's expiration (10).

The same problems of costly expenditures of time, energy, and perseverance exist with the safeguards available to the therapist as with those available to the consumer. There exists the additional ethical dilemma of disclosure and discussion of inadequate treatment resources with a patient who because of his/her illness either cannot fully comprehend the implications of that inadequacy or for whom the knowledge of the inadequacy undermines the treatment.

What other options, then, are available to make sure that allocation decisions take into account more than quantifiable, observable data? There are at least two places or times in which it is crucial to evaluate ethical considerations if, indeed, one believes that they should be regarded at all. The initial discussion stage in which services or care would be discussed would seem to be a logical first place. Although currently there is discussion about the implications of the choice of treatment or length of care, these discussions do not appear to deal squarely with ethical implications. Discussion of ethical considerations might involve the balancing of costs with the accessibility of equitable health care to the poor. Discussion might include the balancing of societal obligations with individual responsibility to make sure that adequate levels of care are available without excessive or disproportionate burden to the individual. Lastly, such a discussion at the early stage of allocation decisions might serve to *not* limit the attainment of equitable access for those least able to pay by providing an alternative focus to discussions about maintaining a "lid" on rising health care costs. Thus, ethical considerations and principles could serve the valuable purpose of providing a counterbalance for decisions otherwise made solely on the basis of fiscal expediency.

A second assessment place might be at certain predetermined intervals after a health program had been determined and treatment plans had been in use for a certain amount of time. Concurrent documentation by the treatment facility and therapist of the effect of certain HMO provisions would then be available to the HMO board along with patient/consumer (individuals or groups) participation. These discussions would not only look at the documented effects of the provisions in question but would also provide a forum for ethical principles to be raised and discussed in the context of the very real consequences as observed by those participating in the HMO (therapist and patient/consumer). Again, this might allow for changes, deletions, or modifications that would bypass the more lengthy process of external review. Nonetheless, one could create an *external* review administrative agency whose charge it would be to monitor HMO health care delivery. We believe that this would, in turn, add a panoply of administrative ills such as we have witnessed with the Environmental Protection Agency (EPA).

Therefore, we believe that a more expedient and indeed more humane proposal would be to provide and maintain an *internal* system of review. This review would provide for discussion of ethical principles to occur at both the initial decision-making stage and predetermined intervals. In many ways this could be comparable to the Institutional Review Boards (IRBs) created to monitor the balance of individual risks with potential research gains. Both IRBs and our proposed review process must include representatives from the participating groups. For HMO review this would seem to include members from the HMO board, therapists, patients, and their advocates. Such an internal review board, we feel, offers the best hope of allocating finite health care resources while retaining sensitivity toward humanitarian concerns.

CONCLUSIONS

In summary, we remain pessimistic about a just societal distribution of mental health care resources. Nevertheless, we do not advocate inaction. We feel that the present economic changes in mental health care must call forth from both provider and consumer renewed concern and energy for an equitable distribution of resources. This we believe is most likely to be achieved by consumer and provider working together in ways that need not involve the congested, expensive, and time-consuming legal system.

ACKNOWLEDGMENTS

Preparation of this paper was supported by the Veterans Administration Research Service. The authors thank Professor Daniel Wikler of the Department of Philosophy, University of Wisconsin–Madison, for comments and review of this manuscript.

The views expressed in this manuscript are those of the authors. They do not necessarily reflect the views and policies of the state of Wisconsin or the Veterans Administration.

REFERENCES

1. Long, F. A. (1984). Federal R & D budget: Guns versus butter. *Science, 223,* 1133.
2. U.S. Department of Commerce. Federal Outlays for Health (#152). *National Statistical Abstract of the U.S. 104th ed.* Washington, DC: Author.
3. President's Commission for the Study of Ethical Problems in Medicine and Biomedical and Behavioral Research. (1983). *Securing access to health care* (Vol. One Report). Washington, DC: U.S. Government Printing Office.
4. Mill, J. S. (1957). *Utilitarianism.* Indianapolis and New York: The Bobbs-Merrill Company. (Original work published 1910).
5. Rawls, J. (1971). *A Theory of justice.* Cambridge: Harvard University Press.
6. Sifneos, P. E. (1979). *Short-term dynamic psychotherapy.* New York: Plenum Publishing.
7. Grimaldi, P. L., & Micheletti, J. A. (1983). *Diagnosis related groups— A practitioner's guide.* Chicago: Pluribus Press.
8. Personal observation, Madison, WI, 1985.
9. Personal observation, San Jose, CA, 1972.
10. Unpublished observation.

10

Accountability and Implications for Supervision and Future Training

Timothy J. Gallagher

INTRODUCTION

The mental health field has come under fire in recent years. It "is being asked to produce more with fewer dollars, to give bigger mental health bang for the buck"(Alger, 1980, p. 391). For more than a decade, the federal government has debated the need for and the role of federal involvement in the training of mental health providers (VandenBos & Stapp, 1983). New burdens on society, including the numerous Vietnam veterans who need help with psychiatric problems, the aging American society with its many elderly who are trying to find their niche, the increasing ethnic minority populations, and the strained American family and concurrent social decay, team with the inflation rate, unemployment, and low economic productivity to produce a major emphasis upon accountability in professions like psychology that are extremely vulnerable to economic cutbacks (Alger, 1980).

Certainly, the state of society has dictated that a new and closer look be taken at mental health care. As resources shrink, third-party payment systems become more prevalent; and as consumers become more aware, the efficacy of psychosocial treatment becomes an important issue. Efficient treatment, measured in terms of dollars and days, begins to intrude upon psychological practice (Alger, 1980). Frank (1979) reports that economic pressures have been exerted on various agencies, resulting in extensive staff cutbacks. As a result, the manner of client treatment has been changed from largely individual sessions in the evenings to primarily group treatment. Length of treatment has also been affected. There has emerged a greater emphasis on limiting treatment to three-to-six-month periods, and group and family treatment modalities are also emerging. Evaluations have focused on trying to find new ways to increase efficacy, to standardize practice, and to eliminate wasted money in the training and distribution of mental health providers (VandenBos & Batchelor, 1983).

The General Medical Education National Advisory Committee reports that increased attention has been devoted in recent years to both the oversupply and undersupply of specific mental health professionals and to assessing the range and appropriateness of their preparation in specific areas (General Medical Education National Advisory Committee, 1980). Other federal agencies have examined both the manner of distribution of mental health providers (Alcohol, Drug Abuse, and Mental Health Administration, 1978) and society's requirements for mental health professionals and specialties (Government Accounting Office, 1984); they have found need for improvement in all areas.

In the face of growing accountability concerns in all areas of society (Alger, 1980), an important facet of training programs for human service providers must include a concern for the monitoring of the quality and effectiveness of care.

In part, the past variability in training and preparation of mental health care providers lies in the disparity in education philosophy. At present, there is "an ever increasing growth of theory on the one hand, and an almost explosive expansion of 'schools of practice' on the other" (Frank, 1979, p. 392). Such divergence between theory and practice has been a source of disunity in the profession and has prevented a more efficient development of available human resources. The professional schools, such as the California School of Professional Psychology, have become more popular because they stress the importance of combining theory, research, and practice and manage more efficiently to train skilled practitioners.

Education is extremely important in providing the balance between theory and practice at the point of entry into the profession. Theory provides a necessary foundation in professional thinking, but new technology and the move toward decentralization point to hands-on experience as the more efficient way of acquiring professional skills. Such techniques as observation, experience through internship, and modeling in the form of faculty demonstration and video presentation seem to be the more valuable approaches from an efficiency standpoint. In the teaching of counseling/interviewing skills, although no standard procedure is defined, "some kind of model, or component of a model, and often the opportunity to practice" is included (O'Toole, 1979, p. 419).

Rogers (1984) offers another view of the current problem and indicts the mental health establishment for its failure to encourage experience among students: "If they really wanted to turn out psychologists capable of independent thinking, they would give them much more freedom and much more opportunity to help form their own curriculum and decide their own goals and use more self-evaluation and so on . . . I think much of our graduate training has as one of its major by-products the damaging of a person's self-confidence (Rogers, 1984).

SUPERVISION AND ITS ROLE IN TRAINING

To learn more effectively in the hands-on situation, including learning to think independently and in new and far-sighted ways, however, requires that greater attention be turned to supervision. It is through effective supervision that practitioners come to acquire the knowledge and variety of skills they need in order to be most valuable to the greatest range of clients, as well as the professionalism to know when expert referrals are needed and where to make such referrals. Herbert Pardes, director of the National Institute of Mental Health, noted in 1983 that of particular concern to the NIMH in the area of training of personnel is the shortage of funds to support students in psychology and social work and the relief of service-delivery obligations for psychiatry faculty so that they can have time for teaching and supervision (Pardes, 1983, p. 1359).

Beyond simple demographics, the needs for future training in current thought focus on the *quality* and *style* of supervision. Giving feedback to trainees regarding their personal and professional behavior is a highly important part of counselor training programs and remains fundamental to the phenomenon of learning (Bernstein & Lecomte, 1979; Worthington & Roehlke, 1979). At its most basic, supervision involves "two individuals, the supervisor and the supervisee, interacting with each other" (Hess, 1980, p. 15). This stipulation applies whether the area of concern is supervision in teaching or supervision in psychotherapy.

One firm definition of supervision dominates the literature and, as Loganbill and associates (1982) observed, the term is often widely applied to pure technical administrative supervision, to beginning skill training, and to the intense therapeutic process. The most concise and accurate definition of supervision appears to be that of supervision as an "intensive, interpersonally focused, one-to-one relationship in which one person is designated to facilitate the development of therapeutic competence in the other person" (Loganbill et al. 1982, p. 4). As Hess (1980, p. 16) states, "supervision is essentially a dyadic human interaction with a focus on modifying the behavior of the supervisee, so he or she may provide better service to a third person (patient) not ordinarily present. . . ."

In addition, the trainee's knowledge of theoretical concepts, concrete skills, and highly personal reaction to the client must also be integrated in the process of supervision (Loganbill et al., 1982). Thus, of the four primary functions of supervision, the most imperative is ensuring the welfare of the client, while the other three are tied to enhancing the abilities of the supervisee.

There are distinct advantages of the clinical supervision model over normal teaching approaches or on-the-job training. Clinical supervision is based on an understanding between the supervisor and the supervisee that their relationship is mutual and that their relationship is one of colleagues and not of superior/subordinate. It is a phase of instructional supervision that draws data from the firsthand observation of actual teaching events and firm face-to-face interaction between the supervisor and supervisee in the analysis of teaching behaviors and activities for instructional improvements (Goldhammer, 1969).

In general, all supervision models have similar content and include the following:

1. Establishing the supervisor/supervisee relationship;
2. Agreeing on the focus of the observations;
3. Observing and collecting descriptive data;
4. Analyzing the data;
5. Discussing the meaning and implications that the data hold for the behavior of the supervisee; and
6. Planning for long-term development and future observations.

The task of supervision in these times of greater accountability is to cover all of this ground with the supervisee as efficiently as possible, while promoting self-motivation, confidence, independent thinking, and a systems viewpoint.

Proponents of clinical supervision argue that if instructional improvement in the classroom is the ultimate goal of supervision, then the supervisor must be willing to spend considerable time working with individual teachers on classroom problems or issues. Therefore, whatever the supervisor's individual style, the supervisor must have superior planning, data-collecting, analysis, and human-relations skills (Goldhammer, 1969).

In supervision in psychotherapy training, six approaches have been identified, all of which have implications for future training needs across the human service professions: *lecturer, teacher, case review, collegial–peer, monitor,* and *therapist* (Hess, 1980). The lecturer approach is one sided and places the supervisor in the role of master to an audience of disciples; global concepts are conveyed and techniques are imparted, but the relationship is essentially unequal. In the teacher approach, the relationship is that of superordinate to subordinate, and specific content and skill are taught within a programmed scheme. Similarly in the case review approach, the more experienced practitioner guides the less experienced practitioner in ways of thinking and relating to cases. The collegial–peer approach works from the basis of the two participants as equal in the relationship; the emphasis is on support and on gaining a different but evolving view.

The monitor approach places the supervisor in the role of an external censor and evaluator who is charged with the duty of maintaining "at least minimally acceptable levels of service" (Hess, 1980, pp. 16–25). The supervisor role is benign in the therapist approach, as the supervisor strives to help the psychotherapist to grow and to increase in the ability to adapt.

For the kinds of professionals needed in the coming decades, the lecturer, teacher, monitor, and to some extent the case review approaches should become less prevalent, as they do not promote the independent thinking of the supervisee. Approaches that require more energy and promote a collaborative, flexible, and adaptive professional will flourish.

Two functions of supervision are teaching and testing, and the models that emerge from these functions are largely dependent upon the theoretical orientation of the supervisor (Moldawsky, 1980). The following sections of this chapter will discuss supervisory models that have implications for the future training of mental health professionals; these include the developmental, behavioral, psychodynamic, interpersonal-process-recall, and structural models. The reasons for this discussion are twofold: (1) Accountability of field education requires clear and purposeful models of supervision and (2) future training needs suggest that a recombining of various current theoretical approaches to supervision may better prepare professionals for their emerging new roles.

The *developmental model* has been popular among many who deal with the training of mental health care providers. Based upon thinking and research in the field of developmental psychology, it emphasizes the profound respect for and belief in the inner capabilities of the individual (Loganbill et al., 1982, p. 14).

The most thorough discussion of counselor training and supervision as a developmental process arising from the changing needs of the supervisee has emerged from Hogan, who views counselors in training as struggling "from an anxious, dependent, method-bound, naive stance through an often painful process of skill acquisition and self-discovery" (Reising & Daniels, 1983, p. 236).

Hogan recommends that supervisors assist supervisees in gaining more accurate perceptions of clients, supervisors, and the self through teaching, support, modeling, and awareness; ambivalence clarification; active confrontation; sharing and supervisee encouragement. In essence, under Hogan's developmental model, a structure emerges to take the supervisee from novice to master and to identify each task in the developmental stage (Reising & Daniels, 1983, p. 236).

Loganbill and associates (1982) also profess a developmental model of supervision, and make three basic assumptions about the process. The first and most obvious assumption is that "core concepts in developmental theory apply to the development of the counselor/therapist" (p. 15). Further, they assume that "distinct stages in the development of the counselor/therapist exist" and that these exist in "definite sequential order." The final assumption is that growth both within and between developmental stages occurs in "a careful sequence of experience and reflection" (p. 15). These assumptions form the basis of the three stages of supervisee development they consider important to the developmental model of supervision: stagnation, confusion, and integration.

This model of supervision is important to acquiring adaptive skills and avoiding professional stagnation because it views supervisee development as being continuous and ongoing; it makes a strong case for continued education and retraining for all mental health professionals, proposing that these stages be gone through over and over again "with each issue receiving greater thoroughness" (Loganbill et al., 1982, p. 17). There are eight issues critical to the supervision process: competence, emotional awareness, autonomy, identity, respect for individual differences, purpose and direction, personal motivation, and professional ethics. All are fundamental to the existence of competent professionals, in the future as well as the present.

A different methodology is exhibited in the training and supervision of behavior therapists. Linehan (1980) stresses that "The basic goals of therapy supervision, regardless of therapeutic orientation, are to assist the therapist both to do effective therapy in the present and to achieve the capability to carry out effective therapy independent of the supervisor" (p. 149). As she points out, models of therapy have been the underlying basis for the development of methods of psychotherapy supervision and ". . . it is more likely that supervisors will employ a model of supervision similar to their own model of therapy" (p. 149).

The *behavioral model* of supervision emphasizes the teaching of a scientific, behaviorally oriented conceptual approach. Linehan (1980) points out several behavior models of supervision, ranging from those that stress the consultative role of the behavior therapist, to the behaviorally taught practicum with stress on consultation and treatment skills, to the systems approach. Underlying the recommended three-dimensional model of behavioral supervision that Linehan herself (1980) recommends is a tripartite model of human functioning that "suggests that behavior can be fruitfully conceptualized as occurring in one or more response systems: the cognitive system (thinking), the overt motor system (actions), and the physiological/affective system (feelings)" (p. 176).

The behavioral model is seen as being most applicable to the goals of supervision, and the skills required by the behavior therapist determine procedures and evaluation of the supervision process (Linehan, 1980). In short, the behavioral model of supervision professes that "one of the most important tasks of supervision is teaching trainees to look to their clients' behavior instead of to the supervisor of clinical theory for validation of their skill" (Linehan, 1980, p. 177).

This, of course, is exactly what current ideals of accountability demand: The process must be of value to the client or it is by definition not valuable. For this reason, it is likely that the behavioral model of supervision will play a very important role in the future training of psychotherapists.

The *psychodynamic model* of supervision places emphasis on the adoption of an analytic attitude which demands that the therapist respect the patient's autonomy, exhibit a genuine and warm interest in the patient, recognize the resistance within the patient, and remain emphatic yet neutral in regard to patient conflicts (Moldawsky, 1980, p. 127). It is the role of the supervisor in the psychodynamic model of supervision to teach the appropriate analytic attitude. Once this attitude has been developed, the transference issue can be handled.

This model of supervision requires that a "learning alliance" be formed between the supervisor and the supervisee. As Moldawsky (1980, p. 131) observes, ". . . therapists often believe in supervision in the same way the patient behaves in therapy. Thus, if a patient is experiencing a sense of helplessness and 'leans' on the therapist, the same sense of helplessness will be reflected in the therapist as he 'leans' on the supervisor." This parallel process becomes an issue to be dealt with in the psychodynamic model.

Four areas have been identified as critical to the psychodynamic supervision experience: teaching, modeling, support, and judgment. It is also the charge of the supervisor to provide means for supervisees to be able to distinguish between supportive psychotherapy and intensive analytic therapy. Moldawsky (1980, p. 134) asserts that "the pleasure of supervision is . . . the gratification that any other teacher or parent receives as the student grows and identifies with the supervisor." The emphasis and concern in the psychodynamic model of supervision is, however, on remaining careful that the supervisee is always a free agent.

The individual as independent free agent is the idea from this model that is most valuable for future training.

The *interpersonal-process-recall (IPR) model* is another approach to training and supervision, designed to provide a method by which mental health professionals can learn and improve their ability to interview, communicate with, and help others (Kagan, 1980). As treatment and supervision efficacy and the team approach to solving problems with appropriate use of shared resources become the *sine qua non* in the mental health care field, the IPR model will perhaps be more important for the future than any other model.

The IPR model consists primarily of a series of interpersonal tasks assessed as necessary for the supervisee to accomplish "in order to obtain knowledge and skill at influencing human interaction" (Kagan, 1980, p. 263). The tasks are sequenced to allow a progression of learning from a least threatening to most threatening phase. When the model is evaluated in relation to traditional supervision practice, significant differences have been observed to emerge regarding counselor behaviors in such categories as "affective," "understanding," "specific," "exploratory," and "effective" (Kagan, 1980, p. 267). Evaluators have found that only a few hours of IPR training are needed before supervisors may be assigned to groups.

Researchers have also found that IPR training results in greater strides with clients. Controlled simulation studies have shown the model to more reliably enable students to make significantly greater gains than control students who received more didactic training. "An additional and unexpected finding has been that the IPR model of supervision is useful in assisting paraprofessionals to learn basic counseling skills" (Kagan, 1980).

The success of the IPR training model lies in its recognition of the need to initiate supervision with attention to skill definition and skill practice, before initiation of intimate interpersonal encounter. In addition to recognizing skills, however, the model also introduces new behaviors that can be considered, learned, and used in nonthreatening ways, such as in film simulation and videotape feedback, in the effort to further reduce anxiety. The individual is also encouraged to make explicit observations regarding perceptions, aspirations, thoughts, and feelings as a part of the process of sharing fears (Kagan, 1980).

The film simulation technique that underlies IPR has given supervision experts great hope for expanded success in the future, but the current process is limited in its implementation because of the lack of a practical and economical procedure. Efforts to continue to refine the model are continuing, however, because work until now has shown that the recall format of the model is valuable in aiding individuals in overcoming their fears and in shortening interpersonal distancing.

Consideration of another mode of intervention, classroom supervision, involves the *structural model* of supervision. A frequently employed technique, it consists of a five-stage sequence of clinical supervision. Supervision under this model ". . . is intended to increase teachers' incentives and skills for self-supervision and for supervising their professional colleagues" (Goldhammer, 1969, p. 55). In addition, this model aims to make the supervision more productive as the teacher increases in teaching skill and professional knowledge. The model is most germane to the teaching setting, so it focuses on the supervisor and the supervisee-as-teacher. For this reason, the teacher's plans are highly important to both parties in the process. The frame of reference of the teacher/supervisee must be made clear "for helping him to function successfully *in his own terms* or for modifying his plans according to concepts existing in the supervisor's frame of reference" (Goldhammer, 1969, p. 58).

In the first stage of the structural model, the supervisee rehearses his plans for teaching, makes revisions to these plans, and reaches an explicit agreement with the supervisor regarding the justification for the supervision in the situation and the manner in which such supervision will occur. In brief, the supervisor and the supervisee create a contract that will determine

the "basis and orientation of the teacher's professional development and for the supervision intended to facilitate it" (Goldhammer, 1969, p. 61).

The second stage of the structural model relates to the ra-
tionale and purpose of the observation. In this stage, the supervisor watches and records the technique and interaction of the
supervisee in his teaching. Such data as emerge are useful in
solving problems of practice and may be used to allow the
supervisee to "test 'reality' by ascertaining whether [the] supervisor's observations . . . tend to confirm or to oppose his own"
(Goldhammer, 1969, p. 63).

Stage three of the structural model deals with analysis and
the creation of strategy to plan the management of the supervision experience. This stage is intended to provide both technical
and process outcomes and to allow the supervisee to learn to
develop his own strategies for practice. An operational plan for
supervision emerges in stage four that culminates in the post-
mortem stage five. The final stage permits the supervisor to
examine his own practice and represents a basis for assessing
whether supervision is working productively and for assessing
its strengths and weaknesses with the aim of modifying supervisory technique accordingly.

The structural model asserts that both the supervisor and the
supervisee are subject to supervision, and to continued education and training. As a result, this model "incorporates supervision of supervision as well as supervision of teaching" (Goldhammer, 1969, p. 72).

The emphasis placed on outcome as assessment of value again
makes this model an important one. Data collection, reality
testing, and strategy creation allow development of independent thinking and a planning orientation that are imperative for
necessary intervention at system levels, skills that true professionals will be unable to be without.

THE ROLE OF EVALUATION

Evaluation is a vital aspect in the training of personnel in all
fields, and many practitioners assert that "evaluation should be
conducted by individuals trained specifically in [the] evaluation
of mental health programs" (Franco & Croft, 1982, p. 1217). As

the mental health care sector acts increasingly like the business sector, evaluation of performance will become increasingly important as a way to determine efficacy, i.e., accountability. In this vein, *performance appraisal* has been found to be a viable method of effecting motivation (Lefton, Buzzotta, Sherberg, & Karraker, 1977).

This model of supervision is primarily concerned with creating a structure in which a formal discussion between a superior and a subordinate occurs for the purpose of determining "how and why the subordinate is presently performing on the job." It is further concerned with assessing how the subordinate may be guided to more effective performance in the future with the aim of benefiting all involved in the process: superior, subordinate, and client (Lefton et al., 1977).

Performance appraisal is a dynamic process that has been found to produce continuous advances in training, even while it differs from other common means of evaluation in its approach to providing subordinates with feedback regarding their performance.

One common approach to providing subordinates with information regarding their performance, ordinary feedback, is "the day-in, day-out commentary that every superior offers his subordinates" (Lefton et al., 1977, p. 7). While such feedback is mainly developmental, it is also casual in that it usually occurs in a spontaneous and unplanned fashion.

A second common approach to evaluation is that of coaching and counseling, which consists of offering analysis of a performance immediately after observation of specific behavior. This approach is primarily a systematic analysis of the performance of a task, and it serves to provide feedback regarding the way in which the task might be better and more efficiently performed in the future.

Performance appraisal differs from these two approaches in several important ways, and it incorporates more extensive goals and results than do the other approaches. Rather than spontaneous feedback, performance appraisal requires that substantial work be undertaken before an appraisal is presented. Data must be gathered and analyzed, and the total performance of the subordinate instead of one specific task, must be considered before an appraisal is offered. Performance appraisal is a carefully considered approach and is not applied on the spot, as with the other two approaches; rather, the procedure usually takes place in the supervisor's office and follows a highly struc- tured, well-organized format (Lefton et al., 1977).

Although this model emerged from the business sector, it provides and incorporates a large amount of expertise that is potentially relevant to training in mental health care. The in- teraction is between the superior and the subordinate (the su- pervisor and the supervisee); the aim is developmental, although the means of modifying performance is behavioral in nature. The psychodynamic concerns of teaching, modeling, support, and judgment should be integrated into this process, and the structural model appears to provide a parallel. In short, performance appraisal seems to be a model that employs the best aspects of the other models reviewed, although the impor- tant aspects of the IPR model are not as evident. A combination of above-discussed aspects of performance appraisal and IPR could form an important and viable model for supervision, given the political, economic, and psychological realities that will exist in the coming years and impinge on the mental health and human services professions.

AFTERWORD

The attention to the training of personnel is only one facet of a more extensive need to scrutinize carefully the contemporary mental health care delivery system. Yet due to the implications it holds for the success of the system, it may well be one of the most important considerations to which attention must turn.

Implicit in this concern is more than the competence of pro- fessionals. Ethical conflict also emerges from different training philosophies, including different supervision and evaluation philosophies. One important area of conflict is the disparity that exists between clinical psychologists and other mental health workers in regard to the medical model. "Such attitudes would seem to lead professionals such as psychologists to experience conflict since they usually work in an arena dominated by pro- ponents of the medical model" (Morrison, Layton, & Newman, 1982, p. 712). A more consistent and evenly balanced approach to training, as well as an understanding of what other pro- fessionals are doing and what they can work together to accomplish with their combinations of skills, might provide the key to defusing this problem and a path into the future. The result would be better and more inclusive services to the most important members of the mental health care community, the clients.

REFERENCES

Alcohol, Drug Abuse, and Mental Health Administration. (1978). *Report of the manpower policy task force.* Washington, DC: U.S. Department of Health, Education and Welfare, Public Health Service, Alcohol, Drug Abuse, and Mental Health Administration.

Alger, I. (1980). Accountability: Human and political dimensions. *American Journal of Orthopsychiatry, 50,* 388–393.

Bernstein, B. L., & Lecomte, C. (1979). Supervisory-type feedback effects: Feedback discrepancy level, trainee psychological differentiation, and immediate responses. *Journal of Counseling Psychology, 26,* 295–303.

Franco, J. N., & Croft, D. B. (1982). Synthesis of training programs for mental health evaluators. *Psychological Reports, 51,* 1211–1217.

Frank, M. G. (1979). Boundaries of theory and practice: Problems in integration. *American Journal of Orthopsychiatry, 49,* 392–396.

General Medical Education National Advisory Committee, U.S. Department of Health and Human Services. (1980). *Summary report of the General Medical Education National Advisory Committee.* (DHHD Publication No. (HRA) 81-651). Washington, DC: U.S. Government Printing Office, 1980.

Goldhammer, R. (1969). *Clinical supervision.* New York: Holt, Rinehart and Winston.

Government Accounting Office. (1984). *Report on mental health manpower.* Washington, DC: U.S. Government Printing Office.

Hart, L. E., & King, G. D. (1979). Selection versus training in the development of professionals. *Journal of Counseling Psychology, 26,* 235–241.

Hess, A. K. (1980). *Psychotherapy supervision.* New York: John Wiley.

Kagan, N. (1980). Influencing human interaction—eighteen years with IPR. In A. K. Hess (Ed.), *Psychotherapy supervision.* New York: John Wiley.

Kramer, J. A., Rappaport, J., & Seidman, E. (1979). Contribution of personal characteristics and interview training to the effectiveness of college student mental health workers. *Journal of Counseling Psychology, 26,* 344–351.

Lefton, R. E., Buzzotta, V. R., Sherberg, M., & Karraker, D. L. (1977). Effective motivation through performance appraisal. New York: John Wiley.

Linehan, M. M. (1980). Supervision of Behavioral Therapy. In A. K. Hess (Ed.) *Psychotherapy Supervision.* New York: John Wiley.

Loganbill, C., Hardy, E., & Delworth, U. (1982). Supervision: A conceptual model. *The Counseling Psychologist, 10,* 3–42.

Moldawsky, S. (1980). Psychoanalytic psychotherapy supervision. In A. K. Hess (Ed.) *Psychotherapy supervision.* New York: John Wiley

Morrison, J. K., Layton, B. D., & Newman, J. (1982). Ethical conflict among clinical psychologists and other mental health workers. *Psychological Reports, 51,* 703–714.

O'Toole, W. M. (1979). Effects of practice and some methodological considerations in training counseling interviewing skills. *Journal of Counseling Psychology, 26,* 419–426.

Pardes, H. (1983). Health manpower policy: A perspective from the National Institute of Mental Health. *American Psychologist, 38,* 1355–1359.

Reising, G. N., & Daniels, M. H. (1983). A study of Hogan's model of counselor development and supervision. *Journal of Counseling Psychology, 30,* 235–244.

Rogers, C. (1984). A new kind of science. *Journal of Counseling and Development, 63.*

VandenBos, G. R., & Batchelor, W. F. (1983). Health personnel requirements, service delivery, and national policy. *American Psychologist, 38,* 1360–1365.

VandenBos, G. R., & Stapp, J. (1983). Service providers in psychology. *American Psychologist, 38,* 1330–1352.

Worthington, E. L., & Roehlke, H. J. (1979). Effective supervision perceived by beginning counselors-in-training. *Journal of Counseling Psychology, 26,* 64–73.

Special Acknowledgment: Barber, N., Bridges, W., O'Neil, J. R., & Mullen, P., for editing assistance.

11

An Ecological Perspective on Behavioral Disorder

Ralph A. Catalano

It has been roughly two decades since the community mental health movement heightened interest in the effect of community dynamics on the incidence, diagnosis, and treatment of behavioral disorder (1, 2). This interest inevitably focused on ecological models that had furthered understanding of behavior in nonhuman communities. Hypotheses inferred from ecological principles appeared in the psychiatric and psychological literature. Many of these hypotheses have been tested and refined or rejected over the last ten to fifteen years. This research is too extensive to review in the space allotted here. I will, rather, go beyond a review and, with considerable trepidation, attempt to infer an ecological perspective on behavioral disorder. I will also briefly describe strategies for prevention that are implied by this perspective.

I will intentionally use "ecological" in a narrower sense than is often found in the psychological literature, in which the term is used to refer to any understanding of behavior that assumes an effect of the social or physical environment. Ecological perspectives are, for my purposes, concerned with communities circumscribed by participation in a trophic organization or energy chain. In human ecology, the trophic organization is usually assumed to be the social organization that develops to convert resources into goods and services. An ecological perspective on behavioral disorder, therefore, would attempt to explain community differences in behavioral disorder as a function of adaptation to change in the means by which we produce and distribute goods and services. These differences can be across communities at one point in time (cross-sectional) or in one community over time (longitudinal).

An ecological perspective on disorder cannot replace traditional psychiatric or psychological explanations of abnormal behavior in individuals. Such a perspective, rather, implies that changes in community organization affect risk factors for disorders that have been identified by research at the individual level. An ecological perspective on disorder should be of interest to psychiatrists and psychologists to the degree they are curious about how the social environment affects the prevalence or incidence of disorder in communities.

ECOLOGICAL CHANGE IN COMMUNITIES

At the risk of oversimplification, it is accurate to say that all ecological models assume a propensity to efficiency. That is, our species is believed constantly to seek ways to increase the yield of goods and services per unit of effort. This belief seems justified, at least in the case of industrial societies, which have universally accepted "economic rationalism" and "scientific management" of one form or another. The propensity to be efficient is most obvious in market economies that are assumed to reward corporate productivity with profits that are passed on to owners seeking personal efficiency through capital investment. Investors are believed to be seeking ventures that will yield returns by introducing products or methods that will make firms or consumers more efficient.

Ecological models further assume that the size and spatial distribution of human communities is determined by a "geometry" of capital investment (3). Every type of productive activity is assumed to be most efficient, and therefore most competitive, at a site or sites that minimize the cost of assembling materials and labor and distributing finished products and services (4). These sites yield communities that expand or contract to the degree that the industries that locate there thrive or decline. A community's size, in other words, is determined by the carrying capacity of its economic base, which, in turn, is fixed by the geometry of capital investment. This belief has generated a long-standing and prolific research tradition that seeks to develop laws that explain historical changes in the spatial distribution of the human population (5). A subset of this work has, in fact, studied the spatial distribution of human disorders (6, 7, 8). Very little work prior to 1960, however, attempted to connect ecological processes with known risk factors for disorder.

Another simplified but essentially accurate inference from ecological models is that the same propensity that leads to the efficient spatial array of population and capital implies a social organization that furthers the efficiency of members. The inputs and outputs of these social machines are often difficult to define, but appear real enough to motivate individuals to participate.

Most, though not all, social organizations are local, in the sense that members are drawn from a geographically circumscribed population. These populations are assumed to be spatially coterminous with communities arising from the geometry of capital investment. Many formal and informal social organizations, moreover, are composed of individuals from the same workplace or industry.

Several corollaries are implied by the above beliefs:

1. The constant search for more efficient production will make the geometry of capital investment very dynamic. Industries, and therefore communities, will become more or less attractive to capital investment as new technologies and competitors change the cost of production and the rate of return.

2. Populations will move in space as individuals seek to maximize personnel efficiency. Communities with stable or contracting economies will require individuals to expend more effort to find secure, rewarding employment than will communities with expanding economies. The relative efficiency of communities in terms of providing secure employment will be manifested in migration patterns that tend to amplify differences in capital investment.

3. Spatial shifts in capital investment and population imply that social organizations are being disrupted. Because social organizations are often geographically based, their membership and functioning are changed significantly by the homeostatic relationship between capital investment and population.

BEHAVIORAL DISORDER IN INDIVIDUALS

Any discussion such as this must inevitably specify the referent for "behavioral disorder." As the term implies, I will mean observable behavior rather than reported discomfort. "Disordered" will mean that the behavior is judged by an audience as sufficiently inappropriate, given the environmental context, that the exhibitor is advised or compelled to seek help. Although this definition will surely not satisfy everyone who considers him- or herself an ecologist, it simplifies conveying an understanding of an ecological perspective on disorder.

As noted above, ecologists have not devised an original explanation of behavioral disorder in individuals but have accepted a model implied by work in several disciplines. This model posits that an individual's risk of exhibiting disordered behavior is a function of three general factors. The first is the degree to which the individual's environment changes and therefore requires behavioral adaptations (9, 10). The second is the ability of the individual to identify and implement appropriate, or socially expected, behavioral responses to changes in the environment (11, 12). The third is audience tolerance for socially unexpected responses (13).

Environmental changes, or stressors, can be further explained as having at least two dimensions, frequency and extent. One could, in other words, experience many or few changes of little or great degree. Many changes of great degree are assumed to require more adaptation than few changes of smaller degree.

The second factor, ability to identify and implement an appropriate adaptation, is assumed to be the product of genetic and acquired skills and propensities. Ecologists accept that the population is composed of good, average, and poor adapters; they assume that the sources of this variation include biological, psychodynamic, and conditioning factors. Determining which of these factors most parsimoniously explains the variation in the population is assumed to be a problem for psychiatry and psychology, not human ecology.

The third construct, audience tolerance, is poorly understood but believed to be a function of two phenomena. The first is the effect of judging the individual's response as disordered on the audience's interests. This is not an easy concept to make operational for many reasons, including the fact that interests are not uniform across any audience, even one as circumscribed as the family. A second component of audience tolerance is the relative power of the audience and the observed. If the latter is much more powerful than the former, he or she is not likely to be affected by audience judgments and may even be able to affect the audience's interests adversely, if an offensive judgment is offered. Powerful audiences (e.g., family or employers), on the other hand, may lead an individual to accept the label of disorder with little resistance.

The above discussion implies the following probability statement that assumes the variables are categorical.

$P_{id} = P_{ifs} \times P_{ie} \times P_{ifg} \times P_{ifa} \times P_{ib} \times P_{ip}$, in which:

P_{id} = probability that individual i will exhibit disordered behavior,

P_{ifs} = probability that individual i will experience frequent stressors,

P_{ie} = probability that individual i will experience stressors of great as opposed to little change,

P_{ifg} = probability that individual i will have few genetic skills to adapt to changes,

P_{ifa} = probability that individual i will have few acquired skills to adapt to changes,

P_{ib} = probability that individual i will exhibit adaptations before an audience that is benefited by a judgment of disorder, and

P_{ip} = probability that individual i will exhibit adaptations before an audience that is powerful enough to affect individual i's fate.

The reason for expressing the assumptions as a probability statement is to emphasize two important points. First, if these categorical conditions were mutually independent, the likelihood of being labeled "disordered" would be, as implied by the statement as written, the product of the separate probabilities. There is, however, good reason to suspect that the conditions are not independent. Persons with little power, for example, are often thought to experience more frequent, if not greater, changes than persons of great power (14, 15).

Second, a community is an aggregate of many individuals who could be represented by a random sample of n persons arrayed in a matrix of *n* rows by seven columns (one for each of the general variables implied by the probability statement). Comparing the matrices of several communities would allow understanding of the sources of variation in the incidence or prevalence of disorder across the communities. The matrix for a community also moves through time. A comparison of the matrices for a community at two points in time would suggest reasons for changes, if any, in the incidence or prevalence of disorder.

CONNECTING ECOLOGICAL CHANGE TO BEHAVIORAL DISORDER

Stressors

Ecological changes impinge on the factors in our probability statement in several ways. The first effect is that the risk of experiencing stressors should vary over time in a community as the industries upon which that community is based become more or less attractive to investors. Communities should also vary cross-sectionally in the risk of participants' being stressed because the industries upon which the communities are based will differ in relative attractiveness. These hypotheses are derived, in part, from the observation that empirically derived lists of stressors include experiences that are related to community dynamics (e.g., loss of job) in addition to those that are associated with a stage in the life cycle (e.g., death of spouse) or that occur randomly (e.g., loss of a pet) (16). Events that can clearly, although not exclusively, be induced by ecological processes can also increase the risk of experiencing other stressors not intuitively associated with community dynamics (e.g., change of residence, change in leisure activities).

Recent research supports the hypothesis that the incidence of stressors will vary longitudinally with shifts in productive activities. Most of this research is cited as support for the belief that economic contraction adversely affects mental health, but the results generalize to the more basic issue of whether ecological processes affect risk factors for behavioral disorder. Shifts in the size (measured in number of employees) of the economic base of a community have been found to be associated with the aggregate incidence of stressful life events (17). More important is the finding that at least the middle class is more likely to experience undesirable job and financial experiences when a region's economy contracts (18). While this association may seem tautological, it should be noted that previous research about stressful life events had not dealt empirically or conceptually with the question of whether stressors over which individuals have little control are randomly experienced or are more likely to occur under social conditions specified *a priori*.

Consistent with the findings of the general research on stressful life events, research on the effect of job and financial stressors reports that such events have a small but significant effect on symptoms (19). The effect is limited to undesirable experiences and survives controlling for socioeconomic and demographic characteristics as well as for all other inventoried stressors. The effect also remains significant when panel designs allow control for earlier symptom levels (20).

Adaptation Skills

Ecological processes are assumed to affect adaptation skills in the short run by taxing the limited ability to adapt. As noted above, ecological research does not intend to replace psychiatric and psychological research that has historically specified the biologic, psychodynamic, and conditioning phenomena that determine how well individuals adapt or respond to environment demands. Some individuals are clearly at such great risk of exhibiting deviant responses for biological or person-based reasons that a consideration of stressors seems academic. Few would argue, however, that most episodes of disorder are unrelated to environmental stimuli. Ecological research has, in fact, been greatly influenced by work most frequently associated with Dubos and Selye that suggests that the quality of adaptation responses is adversely affected by the number of adaptation demands (11, 21). That is, while the capacity to adapt will vary greatly across individuals, that capacity is limited in everyone. Responding to one stressor, therefore, is believed to reduce the capacity remaining to deal with others.

While the fixed-capacity contention is based on biological or cognitive models that are often complex, it can be explained using probabilistic terms. Each of us can be likened to a many-sided die that has a given number of faces that "show" disorder. The proportion of "disordered" faces varies from individual to individual. Stressors are "rolls" of the die in that our audience assess the appropriateness of our response to being stressed. This simile implies two corollaries. First, if all of us are rolled the same number of times, those with the higher proportion of disordered faces are more likely to yield disorder. Second, the best predictor of change in disorder per unit of time for any individual is the number of times he or she is rolled in a time period. The fixed-capacity assumption extends the simile by adding the rule that the proportion of disordered faces goes up with the number of rolls. Depending on the particular version of the model, the increase in disordered faces may start with the first, or come after a threshold number, of rolls and may be a constant or a gradually increasing increment. Variants on the model also specify that the increase has a fixed life, so that the proportion of disordered faces becomes stable if the number of rolls per unit of time remains constant or returns to baseline if the number of rolls decreases.

The importance of the fixed-capacity assumption for an ecological perspective on disorder is that it implies that the stressors inflicted by community dynamics are not only risk factors but may also potentiate or interact with other stressors. Preliminary research on air pollution as a precipitant of psychological distress suggests, for example, that high ozone levels affect symptom levels only among those experiencing other stressors (22). The effect survived controlling for socioeconomic and demographic characteristics as well as for earlier (pre-high-ozone) levels of symptoms.

Audience Tolerance

The suspicion that ecological processes affect tolerance for "out-of-context" behavior arises from a synthesis of work in three fields. The first, and most fully developed, is the sociological literature associated with the social labeling theory of deviance (13, 23). This literature asserts that there is considerable subjectivity in the judgment of which behaviors are disordered. Such judgments are assumed to be influenced by cultural factors that define which behaviors are expected in response to which stimuli, and by the interests and power of the audience. If, for example, a family member behaves in a way that others feel is a threat to the physical, moral, or social well-being of a child (e.g., casual, in-home, use of alcohol), pressure may be brought on the person to modify the behavior or seek help. How likely the person is to seek help depends, at least in part, on the power of the audience to convince him or her that there is a problem that requires action. More important, however, is the implication that the behavior might not have been judged unacceptable by the audience if the family did not include children whose interests were believed to be adversely affected by the drinking. Another implication is that culture and values play a role in defining interests. These factors make judging disorders more subjective than a utilitarian assessment of costs and benefits to a given audience.

The social labeling literature asserts that the behavior of a person who has had an episode of "emotional illness" in the past will be judged by different standards than those applied to the behavior of persons without such a history. Any out-of-context behavior by someone with a previous problem (e.g., "nervous breakdown") is more likely to elicit the judgment of disorder than an identical behavior by others. This phenomenon is believed to lead to the "deviant career" or life-long propensity to seek formal or informal help to reduce the chances of exhibiting behaviors others can exhibit without fear of being labeled disordered (13, 24).

A second literature that has contributed to an ecological view on tolerance is often referred to as "ecological psychology" (25, 26). As the term implies, this field is concerned with the effects of community dynamics on behavior and, therefore, has much in common with human ecology. Ecological psychologists, however, define *community* on a much smaller scale than do human ecologists. The former are most concerned with "behavior settings," which are places that have symbolic meaning derived from the human functions that occur there (e.g., churches, schools, stores). Each type of behavior setting is associated with behaviors that are appropriate there but not necessarily elsewhere. Among the issues ecological psychologists grapple with are how behaviors become associated with settings and under what conditions the associations become stronger or weaker.

One observation associated with ecological psychology is that behavior settings that have more participants than are needed to perform essential functions elicit greater tolerance than those settings with just enough participants to perform the functions. In the latter, or "understaffed," case, participants are claimed to be less judgmental of their colleagues' idiosyncrasies and to tend to have high self-esteem. In the former, or "overstaffed," case, however, participants are described as critical of each other and less confident of their own abilities. The explanation of these effects is that in the overstaffed condition differences supposedly must be found among several qualified persons if only one can be chosen to fill a functional role. The resulting scrutiny leads to finding faults that may or may not affect performance in the role to be filled. In the understaffed condition, on the other hand, participants cannot be critical of each other because survival of the behavior setting requires full participation.

A third literature, which has recently emerged in demography, has also heightened interest in the tolerance construct. This work contends that the social experience and development of an individual is affected by the size of his or her birth cohort (27). This contention has generated several provocative, though largely untested, hypotheses concerning temporal variation in the incidence of behavioral problems. The connection between cohort size and social behavior is assumed to include the heightened competition for resources and positions that members of large cohorts are assumed to experience throughout their life span. This competition is believed to lead to high levels of frustrated aspiration that social scientists have cited as a rising factor for antisocial behavior.

The fourth literature that contributes to an ecological perspective on tolerance is most often associated with organizational management. Classic theories in scientific management posit that firms are machines that include human as well as mechanical components (28). If the overall productivity of the firm is to be maximized, prudent managers must replace less efficient with more efficient machines when the cost of the substitution is less than the value of the added productivity. In the case of labor, one laborer should similarly be replaced by another when the substitution cost is less than the expected gain in productivity. One of the principal strategies of organized labor has been to increase the cost of substitution so that workers will not view themselves as in competition with each other. Labor contracts, therefore, often specify that a person cannot be fired unless management can demonstrate a deficit in an employee's behavior beyond being less efficient than an available replacement.

Several propositions concerning tolerance for out-of-context behavior emerge if the four sets of concepts described above are viewed in the context of community change. The most obvious is that communities that become less attractive to capital investment could experience a period of overstaffing in that natural population increase may not be matched by expansion in opportunities. The perception of this overstaffing may lead persons to become more critical of those seen as competition. Any behavior exhibited by perceived competitors that implies they are inclined to disorder may be cited as reasons to discriminate against them (29).

The lower tolerance possibly engendered by a shift in capital investment may trigger several reactions that lead to an increase in behavior judged as disordered. Persons with histories of "emotional illness," or their families, may sense intensified scrutiny of their behavior and may fear that any indication of a problem will lead to further disadvantage. Behavior not seen as problematic in other persons may, therefore, be judged as "early warnings" that indicate the need for treatment that will preclude more disruptive behavior.

Employees with histories of behavioral problems that affect productivity or work attendance (e.g., alcohol abuse, depression) may be kept when the economy is expanding because the cost of finding a more efficient substitute is high. In an overstaffed labor market, however, efficient persons are found more easily. Management's desire to substitute labor increases and affects the tolerance of work supervisors and families. The individual, his or her family, and management are all on the lookout for behaviors that suggest disorder. The worker and his or her family are looking for early warnings that might allow timely treatment. Management is looking for a reason to allow dismissal "with cause." The result is that behavior that would be tolerated if exhibited at other times is judged disordered.

The above effects on tolerance have been characterized as likely to occur in communities becoming less attractive to capital investment. Becoming more attractive, however, can also reduce tolerance. This is due to the fact that population shifts from communities with stagnant or declining economies to economically growing communities are rarely in proportion to true opportunity. As recent experiences in the Sunbelt demonstrate, there is a tendency for rapidly growing communities to over-attract. This can create the overstaffed, large-cohort effect where least expected.

Research supporting an effect of ecological processes on tolerance has appeared in recent years. Time-series analyses in three different communities have suggested that temporal variation in admissions to mental health facilities is more parsimoniously explained as a function of employment opportunities than of incidence of disorder (30, 31, 32). Research at the individual level, moreover, has indicated that stressors associated with community dynamics increase the likelihood of help-seeking controlling for symptoms and other stressors.

I would also suggest that much of the social support research can be viewed as consistent with the proposition that tolerance affects the likelihood of being judged disordered. Social support is usually seen as a coping resource that mediates the effect of stressors. Persons fortunate enough to have concerned social networks are therefore believed to be at lower risk of responding symptomatically to adaptation demands. The empirical work tends to support this contention and suggests that quality of support is more important than size of social network (33).

The empirical observations in the social support literature can, in my opinion, be parsimoniously explained in ecological terms as a function of the tolerance of the audience. A respondent whose social network is reported to be supportive probably has an audience whose interests are not furthered by judging an out-of-context behavior as disordered. The same behavior exhibited before an audience whose interests are served by such judgment is more likely to be labeled disordered. A respondent in the latter situation is likely to sense the interests of his or her audience and report it to be nonsupportive. Unlike that in the social support literature, an ecological interpretation of the findings suggests further hypotheses as to the conditions under which a social network is likely to be more or less supportive.

Population and Carrying Capacity

Taken together, the above speculations imply that the prevalence of behavioral disorder in communities will vary over time with the ratio of population to carrying capacity. If the economic base expands or contracts such that the population exceeds or falls short of carrying capacity, the risk factors for disorder are affected as follows:

1. The proportion of the population experiencing adaptation demands will increase. The P_{ifs} column of our community matrix will, in other words, show higher probabilities for the individuals in our representative sample.

2. The capacity of the newly stressed individuals to adapt to change will be drawn down. This assumes that at least one of the limited-capacity models of adaptation is accurate and that the average score in the P_{ifa} column of our matrix must become smaller, at least temporarily, as the P_{ifs} scores increase.

3. Tolerance for out-of-context behavior decreases because the social organization has more participants than roles, leading to the overstaffing, large-cohort, or surplus-labor effects. The probabilities of individuals in our sample falling into the P_{ib} category of our matrix, in other words, increases.

The combined effect of the above three shifts is that the average score in our P_{id} column increases, meaning that the prevalence of disordered behavior increases.

IMPLICATIONS FOR PREVENTION

Prevention strategies suggested by the above have been separated into two categories (34). The first, or proactive category, includes attempts to reduce the incidence of stressors through public intervention. Our nation already exercises considerable public control over private investment. These controls include direct regulation as well as fiscal and monetary policies intended to shape the behavior of individuals and firms. Each intervention is assumed to further the general welfare and is implemented after a cost–benefit analysis has been explicitly or implicitly conducted. Most current public policy concerned with the economy is intended to increase productivity by encouraging investment in new plants and businesses. These policies tend to ignore, if not increase, ecologically-induced disorder.

Proactive prevention would be based on a behavioral cost accounting that attempts to estimate the behavioral impacts of policy alternatives. Such an accounting would become part of the cost–benefit analyses that precede policy selection. This added information on costs would, in theory, reduce the likelihood that stress-inducing policies without countervailing benefits would be implemented.

Proactive prevention could also be furthered at the local level. Cities and counties exercise considerable control over private investment through land use and public health codes. These controls could be used to bring carrying capacity and population into balance if behavioral cost accounting were part of the policy formulation process.

The likelihood that behavioral cost accounting will be used in the forseeable future to reduce stressors is not great. This is true for several scientific as well as political reasons. Although research on the behavioral effects of different types of community perturbations is growing, much progress needs to be made before reliable forecasts can inform policy choices. The current societal, indeed international, concern over productivity, moreover, makes public intervention in the private economy to reduce behavioral problems unlikely. It would appear, in fact, that we are on the verge of an era of publicly induced shifts in the geometry of capital investment. Accelerated depreciation schedules, high levels of military spending, and the encouragement of high-tech investment will surely hasten the decline of some and expansion of other communities.

Proactive prevention could also be furthered by increasing tolerance for out-of-context behaviors. This position has been advocated for two decades by those associated with the social labeling school (35). These arguments could become more compelling if the connection between ecological change and tolerance were better understood. This is true because the labeling phenomenon would become an element of the political debate that surrounds the formation of economic policy and the negotiation of labor contracts. The costs of intolerance would therefore become more widely understood and its practice more easily identified and resisted.

A second, or reactive, category of preventions is implied by the recognition that individuals vary in genetic and acquired ability to adapt successfully to stressors. Prevention could be achieved if we better understood how adaptation skills are acquired. Such an understanding could allow teaching individuals at risk of being ecologically stressed to cope more successfully than otherwise would be possible (36). This possibility is exciting in that "stress inoculation" could allow society to hasten ecological change without experiencing the otherwise expected behavioral costs. Such a strategy would be controversial because, among other reasons, it could be viewed as "numbing" or "anaesthetizing" those who are likely to be exploited to increase economic productivity. In any case, the scientific problem of developing a stress-inoculation technique needs to be addressed. This problem is more in the realm of traditional psychology and psychiatry than in that associated with ecological perspectives on disorder.

REFERENCES

1. Barton, W., & Sanborn, C. (1977). *An assessment of the community mental health movement.* Lexington, MA: D.C. Heath.
2. Duhl, L. (1963). *The urban condition: People and policy in the metropolis.* New York, Basic Books.
3. Weber, A. (1968). *Theory of industrial location.* Chicago: University of Chicago Press.
4. Berry, B. (1967). *Geography of market centers and retail distribution.* Englewood Cliffs, NJ: Prentice-Hall.
5. Isard, W. (1975). *Introduction to regional science.* Englewood Cliffs, NJ: Prentice-Hall.
6. Shannon, G., & Dever, G. (1974). *Health care delivery: Spatial perspectives.* New York: McGraw-Hill.
7. Levy, L., & Rowitz, L. (1973). *The ecology of mental disorder.* New York: Behavioral Publications.
8. Catalano, R. (1979). *Health, behavior, and the community.* New York: Pergamon.
9. Meyer, A. (1968). *Collected papers of Adolf Meyer.* Baltimore, MD: Johns Hopkins University Press.
10. Dohrenwend, B. S., & Dohrenwend, B. P. (1976). *Stressful life events: Their nature and effects.* New York: Wiley.
11. Dubos, R. (1965). *Man adapting.* New Haven, CT: Yale University Press.
12. Antonovsky, A. (1979). *Health, stress, and coping.* San Francisco: Jossey-Bass.
13. Scheff, T. (1964). *Being mentally ill: A sociological theory.* Chicago: Aldine.
14. Myers, J., Lindenthal, J., & Pepper, M. (1976). Social class, life events, and psychiatric symptoms: A longitudinal study. In B. S. Dohrenwend & B. P. Dohrenwend (Eds.), *Stressful life events: Their nature and effects.* (pp. 191–206). New York: Wiley.
15. Liem, G. R., & Liem, J. H. (1978). Social class and mental illness reconsidered: The role of economic stress and social support. *Journal of Health and Social Behavior, 19,* 139–156.
16. Ruch, L. O. (1977). A multidimensional analysis of the concept of life change. *Journal of Health and Social Behavior, 18,* 71–83.
17. Catalano, R., & Dooley, D. (1979). The economy as stressor: A sectoral analysis. *Review of Social Economy, 37,* 175–187.
18. Catalano, R., & Dooley, D. (1983). The health effects of economic instability: A test of the economic stress hypothesis. *Journal of Health and Social Behavior, 24,* 46–60.

19. Dooley, D., & Catalano, R. (in press). Why the economy predicts helpseeking: A test of competing explanations. *Journal of Health and Social Behavior.*
20. Aldwin, C., & Revenson, T. *Vulnerability to economic stress: A test of the provocation and social selection models.* Manuscript submitted for publication.
21. Selye, H. (1952). *The story of the adaptation process.* Montreal: Acta Inc.
22. Evans, G., Jacob, S., Dooley, D., & Catalano, R. *The interaction of air pollution and stressful life events on mental health.* Manuscript submitted for publication.
23. Sarbin, T. (1969). Schizophrenic thinking: A role theoretic analysis. *Journal of Personality, 37,* 190–206.
24. Rosenhan, D. (1973). On being sane in insane places. *Science, 179,* 250–258.
25. Barker, R., Shoggen, P. (1973). *Qualities of community life.* San Francisco: Jossey-Bass.
26. Wicker, A. (1979). *An introduction to ecological psychology.* Belmont, MA: Wadsworth.
27. Easterlin, R. (1980). *Birth and fortune: The impact of numbers on personal welfare.* New York: Basic Books.
28. Perrow, C. (1972). *Complex organizations: A critical essay.* Glenview, IL: Scott-Foresman.
29. Berg, I., & Hughes, M. (1979). Economic circumstances and the entangling web of pathologies. In L. Ferman, & J. Gordus (Eds.), *Mental Health and the Economy* (pp. 15–62). Kalamazoo, MI: Upjohn Institute.
30. Catalano, R., & Dooley, D. (1979). Does economic change provoke or uncover behavioral disorder? A preliminary test. In L. Forman, & J. Gordus (Eds.), *Mental Health and the Economy* (pp. 321–346). Kalamazoo, MI: Upjohn Institute.
31. Catalano, R., Dooley, D., & Jackson, R. (1981). Economic predictors of admissions to mental health facilities in a non-metropolitan community. *Journal of Health and Social Behavior, 22,* 284–298.
32. Catalano, R., Dooley, D., & Jackson, R: Economic provocation or psychological disorder: A reformulation of the time-series tests. Manuscript submitted for publication.
33. Gore, S. (1981). Stress buffering functions of social supports: An appraisal and clarification of research models. In B. S. Dohrenwend, B. P. Dohrenwend (Eds.), *Stressful Life Events and Their Contexts* (pp. 202–222). New York: Prodist.
34. Catalano, R., & Dooley, D. (1980). Economic change in primary prevention. In R. Price, R. F. Ketterer, B. Bader, J. Monahan (Eds), *Prevention Health.* Beverly Hills: Sage.
35. Szaz, T. (1960). The myth of mental illness. *American Psychology, 15,* 113–118.
36. Meichenbaum, D., & Jaremko, M. (1983). *Stress reduction and prevention.* New York: Plenum.

12

The California Mental Health Reform Act of 1985: A Case Study of Policy Reform in the Post-Welfare State

James Hynes

INTRODUCTION

In May 1985, California Governor George Deukmejian signed into law AB 2541, the California Mental Health Reform Act, authored by Assemblyman Bruce Bronzan and Assemblywoman Sunny Mojonnier. The passage of this legislation is significant for a number of reasons. First, and perhaps most important, it represents one state's successful efforts to remedy a set of public mental health and social welfare problems in a politically conservative environment that is seemingly indifferent to such problems. Second, the case of mental health reform in California demonstrates the types of issues interest groups will converge on in order to satisfy their separate and collective needs. This, of course, is nothing new. Interest groups have always been salient components of the political process. What is new, however, is that interest-group politics is eclipsing the role that welfare-state politics formerly held over health and welfare issues. This leads to the third major point of significance of AB 2541. For the foreseeable future, as long as conservative social policy influences prevail, it is critically important for all the actors in the mental health complex—whether they be psychiatrists, psychologists, social workers, researchers, consumers, or others—to act in concert as overlapping interest groups concerned about a humane and effective system of care. The case of AB 2541 demonstrates how three main interest groups (researchers, provider professionals, and consumers) came together into a loosely defined, yet effective, force for mental health reform. The rallying point in AB 2541 was the problem of the homeless mentally ill.

OVERVIEW OF THE PROBLEM

California's homeless mentally ill population has grown significantly in the last twenty years. This problem is the direct outgrowth of a mass exodus from state hospitals, coupled with a steady decline in state expenditure for community mental health. State hospitals housed almost 50,000 patients in 1967; today there are fewer than 5,000. Financial commitment for mental health services by the public sector has dropped precipitously, especially in recent years (see Figure 12.1), while other selected areas of public finance have not suffered as badly under the budget crunches (see Figure 12.2).

The homeless mentally ill population is composed of two distinct groups. First, there are the former state hospital inmates released under the community mental health initiative of the 1960s and 1970s. Second, there is an emerging group of young adults, 20–35 years old, who do not have lengthy histories of state hospitalization, but, instead, have been reliant on local hospital acute beds and limited outpatient and residential services.

Recent estimates place the total number of homeless nationwide at between 60,000 and 100,000. One-third of this number, or 20,000 to 35,000, are thought to be mentally ill. They can be found on the streets and under the bridges of our urban communities. For some cities, such as San Francisco and Los Angeles, the problems of the homeless mentally ill population

Figure 12.1 Per capita change in state support
1977–1985 (in 1977–1978 dollars).

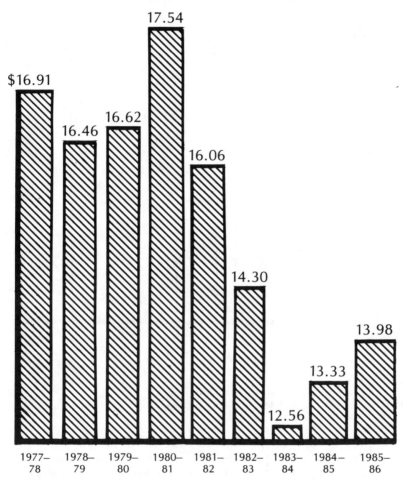

Compiled from data provided by Harry Osborne of the Legislative Analyst's
Office.

are especially acute and have posed troublesome questions of
economics and social control for many city and state officials.
Should they respond by clamping down on civil liberties
through the use of costly institutional settings, or should they
respond by developing new and innovative treatment settings
aimed at basic needs, least restriction, economic feasibility, and
social integration?

Figure 12.2 Percentage change in general
fund allocations 1979–1985 for selected areas.

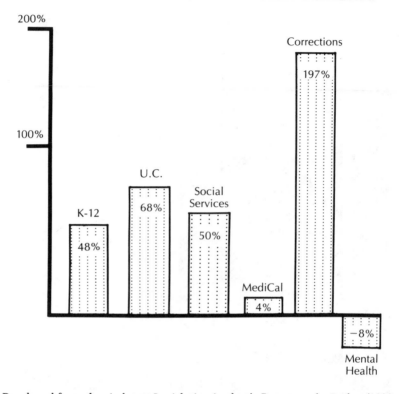

Developed from the six latest Legislative Analyst's *Report on the Budget* (1980–
81 to 1985–86).

At present, 65% of the local mental health budget is used for
treating only 25% of the estimated total number of clients in the
local mental health system. Included in this 65% of Short–Doyle
community monies is the cost for county clients *in state hospital*
beds, the largest expenditure category in the total budget. This
is a questionable way to spend local community mental health
monies. The remaining 75% of the clients receive outpatient
care and/or residential services covered by SSI/SSP, but with
only 35% of the mental health budget.

The governor's recent mental health initiative included budget augmentations for the last two years. These increases are
reflected in the 1984–85 and 1985–86 histograms in Figure 12.1.

Yet there are no guarantees that such augmentations will continue in future years. By definition, the augmentations are temporary and do not signal lasting support to mental health. In fact, as is evident in Figure 12.1, the overall trend is for less support.

The consequences of these past and present spending practices are clear and are well documented in the mental health economics literature. Community treatment alternatives, regardless of the funding source (24-hour care, outpatient, or residential services), have historically been underfunded, and thus, for lack of any other treatment setting, clients end up in a hospital bed or the "street asylum." This is one of the major causative factors behind the so-called revolving door, what one expert testifier referred to recently at a mental health hearing as "a series of psychiatric emergencies treated by hospitalization." The hospital will temporarily stabilize clients, only to release them to the same unsupportive environment they came from. Other causative factors are:

1. 1981 federal actions to terminate thousands of people from their SSI/SSP benefits;
2. The instability of community residential placements, stemming from budget cuts, and the aggressive efforts of facilities to "cream" the population and avoid the difficult clients.

All of the causative factors are highly interactive. The nature of these interactions and the relative importance of each causative factor is not well understood. What is understood, however, are the spending patterns and service categories. These will be expanded on below.

Table 12.1 summarizes 24-hour care expenditures in the following ways:

- costs per bed in different settings,
- total expenditures per service level,
- numbers of beds at each service level.

Over 90% of the budget is used up in local and state hospital expenditures. Local hospital beds, in particular, are the most costly type of 24-hour care bed, at $101,000 per bed per year.

Table 12.1 1982–83 Estimates of Publicly Funded Mental Health Services

	Beds	Total cost ($ millions)	Annual cost per bed
Short–Doyle funded			
State hospital (county patients)	2524	$125.9	$49,872
Local hospital	997	106.0	101,144
Psych. health facility	180	14.0	83,900
Crisis residential	180	5.5	33,000
Transitional care	710	15.3	23,000
Long-term residential	145	3.2	23,500
Out-of-home placements	285	2.4	9,500
Jail inpatient	45	2.3	55,000
SNFs w/ psych prog	—	4.3	NA
MediCal-funded			
Local hospital	427	30.7	71,949
SNFs w/o psych prog	6,500	91.0	14,000

Jail inpatient beds, psychiatric health facility beds, or skilled nursing facility beds with a special psychiatric program are also relatively more costly but represent much smaller percentages of the total expenditure.

Although homeless mentally ill clients may need treatment focused more on basic needs and empowerment, they, too, frequently receive medication and observation in one of the four settings cited above. In fact, clients are given little opportunity to start working on the basic needs of shelter, food, work, and clothes because the very nature of their hospital bed treatment precludes involvement in these areas. The incentives for optimal integration and rehabilitation seem to be reversed.

POLICY BACKGROUND

In recent legislative history, major shifts in California mental health policy occurred in 1957, with the passage of the Short–Doyle Act, and in 1967, with the passage of the Lanterman-Petris-Short Act. Short–Doyle (S-D) established the current state–county *financial* relationship; 90% of a county's community mental health monies come from the state and 10% would come from the county in the form of a matching grant. Lanterman-Petris-Short (L-P-S) established the current *social* relationship between the mentally disabled and the society in which they live. Lanterman-Petris-Short made it much more difficult to carry out civil commitment procedures against someone with an alleged mental illness. Taken together, Lanterman-Petris-Short and Short–Doyle made California's community mental health programs possible. Such programs provided the potential for a cost-effective, humane system of care and assistance—one predicated on the belief in least restriction and maximum integration into society. But, as many in the mental health field now know, this community model of care was only a dream, which was never adequately funded and given a fair chance. And, for at least the immediate future, the trends are for the worse. There is less and less money for communities and a growing indifference to that horde of the "walking wounded," the homeless mentally disabled, those who suffer the consequences of declining mental health monies.

Budget appropriations for community programs dropped throughout the 1970s and 1980s. Some of this resulted directly from federal actions. The Omnibus Reconciliation Act of 1981 set up the block-grant system between the states and the federal government. Mental health was blocked with alcohol and drug programs, with 33% less funding than in the previous year. The act also served to disrupt and weaken existing constituent groups.

At the state level, local community-based programs tended to bear a disproportionately greater amount of the burden of fiscal restraints. The governor's most recent budget proposals have called for redirecting state efforts to the state hospitals, even though hospital services already account for 75% of the total mental health dollar. The governor's 1984–85 budget augmentation called for providing an extra $25 million for hospital programs, but nothing for community programs.

At the local level, Proposition 13, adopted in 1978, greatly curtailed county government spending and, consequently, county ability to provide Short–Doyle matching funds, as required under the Short–Doyle Act. Thus, local program budgets have been getting squeezed at the top by federal cutbacks and at the bottom through the passage of Proposition 13.

It was within this context of legislative and fiscal history that the Select Committee on Mental Health was established.

In November, 1983, Willie Brown, Speaker of the House in the California Legislature, authorized the establishment of the Select Committee on Mental Health. Brown's chief of staff, Steve Thompson; the director of the Assembly Office of Research (AOR), Arthur Bolton; and UC Berkeley public health professor, Leonard Duhl, all played key roles in convincing the Speaker of the tremendous need for a thorough examination of the state mental health system and the experiences of those in it. All three of these people had long histories of involvement in health and mental health policy. Each brought a set of experiences that helped them determine the modes by which legislative change could take place in California mental health. Steve Thompson had worked as a consultant and lobbyist on health policy before his involvement with the Speaker's Office. Leonard Duhl was the former chief of planning at NIMH and had had extensive involvement with the New Frontier and Great Society programs of the Kennedy and Johnson administrations. Arthur Bolton was the chief architect behind the Lanterman-Petris-Short Act and, through his years of experience at AOR, had worked on a broad range of health policy issues. In the few years previous to the establishment of the committee, each one of these people had become acutely aware that health reforms based on liberal-democratic, moral-suasion arguments were becoming increasingly difficult to effect. As Arthur Bolton once remarked, because of the fact that not a single legislative recommendation from AOR was seriously considered by the Republican-dominated legislature and administration, a new strategy had to be developed—a type of guerrilla warfare. In concurring with the need for such a new type of philosophy, Duhl suggested that change, like a stream of water, was inevitable and that any practical efforts at effecting change, or the stream, had to rest more on trying to divert the stream rather than on trying to stop the water. The select committee, as the brain child of Bolton, Thompson, and Duhl, was established in full recognition of this need for a new political strategy.

Select committees differ from standing committees of the legislature in that they are intended to undertake an in-depth, critical examination of a very specific area over a protracted period of time. Based on this critical examination, select committees make recommendations for change, usually in the form of new bills. The intentions behind establishing the Select Committee on Mental Health had much more to do with politics than with policies, programs, and planning. Undoubtedly there was and still is a real desire substantively to evaluate the mental health system, to ask the basic question, "What does the state receive for the half-billion dollars it spends on mental health each year?" This, of course, is an enduring type of question—one that is, or should be, a part of all legislative debates.

In the years previous to the work of the Select Committee on Mental Health, this question was brought up by other legislators, such as Tom Bates. His work resulted in the passage of AB 3052 of 1979, what is now known as the Bates Bill. This bill funded a few programs around the state at levels nearly commensurate with what the Bates legislative work group recommended for an effective, comprehensive, community-based system of mental health care. Unfortunately, support for these programs, however cost-effective they may be, has not been very strong from the Dukmejan administration. Follow-up legislation that would have allowed the growth of more of these programs never occurred, because it simply was not politically viable. Consequently, the case of the Bates Bill represented how legislative change did in fact occur, but without really shaking out the entire system in which change occurred.

In establishing the Select Committee on Mental Health it was hoped that an in-depth, eighteen-month study would be sufficient not only in defining particular mental health problems, but, more importantly, in providing the context in which political interest groups could rally around mental health needs and exert an undeniable political presence.

INTEREST GROUPS AND THEIR AREAS OF CONCERN

Throughout the committee's ten hearings, it became clear that there were at least three major groups in the arena of mental health politics. They were (1) the researchers—mostly biomedical, psychiatric, and academic, (2) the professional providers—clinicians, social workers, and counselors, and (3) the consumers and their families.

As Table 12.2 illustrates, each of these interest groups' concerns varied markedly over the resource areas of facilities, financing and organization, manpower, participation, and research.

The research group concerns were distributed mostly over the areas of facilities and research. Manpower and financing issues were much less of a concern to this group, but were more of a concern to the professional providers and the consumer interest groups. Consumer groups tended to be more concerned with facilities and participation issues. This group did not voice even one concern in research issues. The professional provider interest group tended, in general, to be less extreme on any one resource area, but they were the group which voiced the most concern over manpower, financing, and organization resource areas.

It should be noted that any further analysis would be highly subject to debate. Only half of the hearings of the committee are represented in Table 12.2, and these hearings were not selected randomly; furthermore, the units of analysis in this table are "numbers of recommendations per area per group," which can at times be a purely subjective measure. Any further quantitative analysis may likely lead to spurious conclusions.

However, it is still possible to conduct a qualitative analysis, thus making it possible to continue studying the attitudes of the three interest groups toward various resource areas. Instead of "number of recommendations per area per group" as the unit

Table 12.2 Quantitative Analysis of Major Resource Areas

(Numbers refer to # of recommendations/area/group)

Interest-Group Resource Area	Research	Provider	Consumer	Total
Facilities	20	17	30	67
Financing and Organization	2	9	6	17
Manpower	3	8	6	17
Participation	7	10	16	33
Research	19	4	0	23
Total	51	48	58	157

of analysis, qualitative analysis is based on "who says what about whom, why, when, and where." A qualitative analysis was conducted on half of the hearings by this author, but for the sake of brevity, will not be included here. The format of the analysis is demonstrated in Table 12.3.

Based on this type of qualitative analysis, the committee identified the following areas as the ones needing the most attention by the legislature.

1. Facilities and participation issues affecting the chronically mentally ill. These include self-help, social support, housing and employment, and just basically having the right resource at the right place at the right time.

2. Research, psychosocial and biomedical issues. The committee found that too frequently state-of-the-art advances did not find wide-spread applications at the clinical/practitioner level.

3. Social control issues. The committee was concerned about the definition of "gravely disabled" in the Lanterman-Petris-Short Act. At times the "gravely disabled" criterion was too subjectively interpreted and too often led to either no care at all or inappropriate care for a mentally disabled person.

4. System information and evaluation capability issues. The committee found that information and data resources were not letting us know how services and funding were distributed across the state.

5. Children's mental health issues. The committee found a tremendous amount of uncoordination and confusion about children's mental health resources. Though there are a myriad of agencies for children, the experience of any one child is based more on chance than on a coordinated referral system.

Based on hearing testimony, these are the areas which allowed for the development of interest group alliances. The Committee successfully addressed itself to achieving "win–win solutions" which met large and important areas of real need in mental health services. Yet, despite the Committee's efforts at "win–win solutions," not all of these areas were equally treated in the final set of legislative recommendations contained in AB 2541. Though research concerns were highly endorsed by the research interest group, there simply was not enough support

Table 12.3 Qualitative and Quantitative Analysis of Interest Group Recommendations on "Participation" in the Mental Health System

Interest-Group Resource Area	Research	Provider	Consumer
	(numbers refer to # of recommendations/area/group)		
Participation			
Family	Berger, Greenblatt, and Lamb all support the concept of more family involvement in mental health services and systems. Lamb supports the idea of home-based care. Jamison wants the family better educated about recurrent nature of depression	Levine wants the family included in psychosocial support. Lewis wants family educ. and integration in client social context. Farr agrees.	Harp, Dorsey, and the Davenports emphatically support family involvement in the client's treatment mileau. 10
Community	Greenblatt advocates more community involvement and awareness of mental health issues.	Levine wants more community interaction with mental health clients as a therapy. Lunsford wants better communication with communities. O'Connor believes in CMHC concept. Farr wants the community to be trained.	The Davenports want more community involvement. Harp believes that all efforts must be aimed at the community. Hudson want a "sense of community" and a "comprehensive network of community institutions" to deal with all of our social services. 8
Client Self-Help	Greenblatt and Eisdorfer support efforts at increasing self-help opportunities.	Leavitt, Britter, Ross all support work in areas of self-help with the elderly, adolescents	Harp-"empowerment" as key to self-help. Basics of housing and jobs, gov bds. as start of self-help. Self-determination. Kennedy, Zinman, Williamson want clients as staff. Hudson, Schraber, Shabinski, Cunningham, Kiel, Singer support self-help. 15
TOTAL	7	10	16 33

from other interest groups, most notably, the consumer interest group. On the other hand, researchers endorsed self help and social support facilities, which the consumer interest group heavily endorsed and the professional provider interest group moderately endorsed. Since all three interest groups were in agreement on self help and social support facilities the final set of recommendations specifically covered that. In much the same way that, through the dance of interest group politics, other recommendations of AB 2541 congealed. They came out of uncertainty and confusion about how to go about mental health reform and what to expect from the mental health system of the 1980's.

THE SOCIAL SUPPORT AGENCY RECOMMENDATION OF AB 2541

The budget appropriation for AB 2541 was $53 million dollars over a three-year period. This money was targeted to different areas, including the homeless mentally ill, children's mental health services, mental health in county jails, involuntary outpatient treatment, services for the rural elderly, Vietnam vets, and more.

The social support agency recommendation of AB 2541 constitutes the bulk of the money allocated. It was the one issue that received far more attention from the testifiers, the media, and the administration than any other recommendation.

Since current treatment facilities do not place enough emphasis on the securing of resources to meet the basic needs of clients, such as housing, clothing, jobs, income maintenance, and food, the social support agencies (SSAs) recommendation of AB 2541 was proposed to create better coordination within existing networks of services available. The premise of the recommendation rests on the notion that social, medical, psychological, and other services may already exist in adequate amounts. The goal of the recommendation is to coordinate existing diverse resources to better meet the basic needs of clients. Coordination is to be done by a case manager, a psychology professional knowledgeable on mental health services and finance who is also capable of assisting clients with securing resources to meet their basic needs.

Figure 12.3 outlines agency relationships in terms of dollar flows and accountability (via audit reports). For convenience

Figure 12.3 Organizational relationships between social support agencies (SSAs) and other governmental agencies.

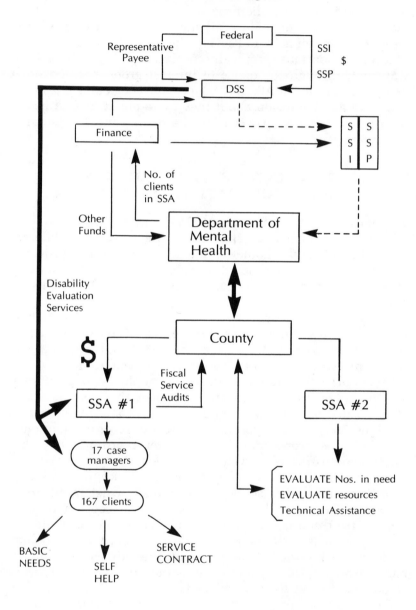

and clarity, only one county and two SSAs are presented, instead of three counties and six SSAs, as specified in the legislation. Each of the SSAs will have a client load of approximately 167 and 17 case managers. In total, there will be 1,000 clients and 100 case managers across all six SSAs. This amounts to a 1 to 10 case manager to client ratio, which is significantly less than the case-loads ratio in the current mental health system. This occurs despite the fact that the SSAs require a funding level per client, from SSI/SSP, of only $10,000 per year.

CONCLUSION

At this writing, counties are just beginning to implement the social support recommendations for the chronically mentally ill homeless. Although it is too early to tell just how effective these programs will be, it is clear that each county is approaching the issue differently. Some counties are developing programs that approach the organization structure outlined in Figure 12.3. Other counties are developing programs of a more modest scope, based on the work of a "housing advocate."

The experiences of these counties should be closely monitored in order to guide future program development in other areas. All of the other recommendations of AB 2541 will need at least another year in operation before they can be realisticly evaluated. As with the social support agency recommendation, the implementation of these recommendations should be closely monitored. Although the committee has been disbanded and its members have moved on to other positions in the legislature, it should be remembered that clean-up legislation based on county experiences with AB 2541 will be in the offing. This is especially true since Assemblyman Bronzan is presently the chair of the Assembly Ways and Means subcommittee on health and welfare.

It appears likely that Governor Deukmejian will be reelected, and thus the administration will continue to exert an anti-welfare state philosophy at the state level. Other than suggesting refurbishment of state hospitals, the governor has not offered any other constructive suggestions or reforms in mental health. This certainly means that current and future reform efforts must derive from collaboration among mental health interest groups. They must work together at defining leverage points where their mutual interests converge, just as occurred with the homeless mentally ill. Any other efforts at broad-based reforms will ultimately fail and may, in fact, cause more harm than good. It has been the hope of this chapter to inform all of the actors in the mental health complex of the conditions at the policy development level that affect their work and through which they can effect change.

REFERENCES

Auditor General of California. (1985). *The state's mental health system could be operated more cost-effectively and could better meet the needs of clients.* Sacramento: Office of The Auditor General.

Blum, H. (1981). *Planning for health: Generics for the eighties.* New York: Human Sciences Press.

Janowitz, I. (1965). *Social control of the welfare state.* New York: Academic Press.

Kiesler, C. (1982). Public and professional myths about mental hospitalization. *American Psychologist, 37,* 1323–1339.

Office of The Legislative Analyst. (1984, March). *Report on the public mental health system.* Sacramento: Author.

Robertson, M., & Ropers, R. (1985). *Basic shelter research project (Document #4).* Los Angeles: UCLA, School of Public Health.

Epilogue

The viewpoints of the expert contributors to this volume are not intended to be solutions. They are simply sketching out the parameters of the shapers on the field. We have touched upon the demographic, economic, political, research, and business issues of mental health in the mid-1980s. These issues will wax in importance over the next few decades and form the basis for a new dialogue among the actors within the mental health complex.

As we look to the future, we must continue to develop better dialogue among the rather heterogeneous set of actors in the mental health field. Collaboration and dialogue must characterize our approach to the problems of dwindling resources, cost-containment arguments, and fewer and poorer services. Without dialogue it may be impossible for any of us to work effectively in the field. Dialogue is of the upmost importance as we develop new paradigms and ways of thinking that go beyond narrow professional concerns.

Even more important, however, is the role of the consumer groups. Although we have been focusing on the systems issues, the greater issues reside in the needs of our clients, patients, and the population at large. We cannot ignore the poor, the homeless, the middle class, or even the rich. They are part of the future, and the future is now.

To participate in the emerging world, we must all act now.

We must begin to encourage mental health consumers to take the actions necessary for them to learn how to manage their lives. As a consumer of mental health services, Howie Harp has suggested that future programs, in light of all the cost containment arguments, should be client-run as volunteers and staff who provide effective role models—people who have been in hospitals and know what it is like first hand to "make it on the outside."

Types of self-help groups include, but are not limited to:

- Peer Support Groups: very effective, requiring little or no funding.
- Independent Living Programs: adapting a proven, effective model of deinstitutionalization for mental health clients, e.g., The Mental Disabilities Independent Living Project.
- Drop-in Centers: providing socialization and support, membership-run volunteer programs, as were pilot programs in New York and Florida.
- "Friendly Visitor" Programs: visiting members at home and hospitals such as the "Reach Out Committees" in Oakland.
- Performing Groups: using drama to improve conditions and themselves, such as "We Can Players" in Riverside, CA.
- Other groups: including *businesses* and *advocacy groups*.

Recognizing the great significance of these words, we must rethink our roles. As the Communications Era Task Force recently pointed out, our future roles may be that of "communicators of skills and techniques" rather than solely that of a direct service provider. Again, *dialogue* is the most important factor that should guide our future roles. The clients' involvement in the dialogue is essential. Without communication from them, many of our mistakes of the past will be repeated. Many of the professionals in the mental health complex must be mindful of this as their roles shift in the changing sociopolitical environment. It is for this reason that the two editors, each with many years experience in their own and related disciplines, came together to put forth a call for action. It is time!!

Index

Index

Abuse, in children, 37–38
Acquired immune deficiency
 syndrome (AIDS), NIMH
 research and approaches
 addressing, 43–44
Adaptability
 behavioral disorders and,
  139–140
 mental well-being and, 16
Adapters, in population, 136
Agent Orange, 24–25
Aging
 of America, 19, 20
 health care in, 22–23, 38–39
Alcohol abuse, *see* Substance
 abuse
Alcohol, Drug Abuse, and Mental
 Health Administration
 (ADAMHA), 31
Alternative health care
 paradigms of, 6
 of serious mental disorder,
  65
Antisocial behavior, *see also*
 Crime
 perceptions of, 23
Audience tolerance
 behavioral disorders and,
  140–144

business management issues
 and, 143
ecological processes in, 143–
 144
explanation of, 136–137

Bandura, A., 62
Bates, T., 157
Behavioral cost accounting, use
 of, 146
Behavioral disorder
 connecting ecological change
  to, 138–145
 definition of, 136
 ecological perspective on,
  133–148
 in individuals, 136–138
 model of, 136
 population and carrying
  capacity in, 144–145
 prevention of, implications for,
  145–146
 probability statement on,
  137–138
Behavioral model of supervision, description of, 123–
 124
Beutler, L. B., 101–102
Bias

Omnibus Reconciliation Act of
1981, effect of, 42, 155
Organizational management,
tolerance and, 142–143
Out-of-context behavior, tolerance and, 140–141, 143, 146

"Para" societies, development of,
9–10
Performance appraisal
comparison of, with other
evaluation techniques,
128–129
use of, 128
Personality characteristics, of
mental health professionals,
57–58
Perspective, common biases of,
62–64
Physician-patient ratio, in US,
86–87
Politics, in mental health care,
7–8
Population and carrying capacity, relationship of, 144–145
Population changes, in US, 19–21
Preferred provider organizations
(PPO)
description of, 88
growth of, 48–49
impact of, 49–50, 52
mental health and, 89
Prevention research, in mental
health care, 41
Private practice, endangerment
of, 85
Proactive prevention techniques,
behavioral disorders and,
145–146
Professional organizations, properties and processes of, 56–
57
Provider groups, mental health
interests and concerns of,
158–161

Psychiatric utilization rate, inpatient, by HMO members,
80
Psychiatrists
personality characteristics in,
57–58
as physicians, 58–59
professional perspective of,
58–59
Psychiatry, medicalization of, 5,
61
Psychodynamic supervision experience
approaches to, 121–122
models of, 122–127
Psychoimmunology, 5
Psychological thought, in mental
health, 6
Psychological trauma, sequelae
of, 38
Psychologists
clinical vs. scientific, 59–60
insurance plans and, 61
professional perspective of,
59–60
Psychology, accountability in,
117
Psychosocial thought, mental
health field and, 6–7
Psychosocial treatment, efficacy
of, implications of, 118
Psychotherapeutic knowledge,
codification of, 103
Psychotherapy
consumer-driven vs. provider
controlled, 104
in the future, 99
issues in, 99–100
qualifications to do, 99–101
strategies for, 100
Public interest, in advocacy for
mental health in HMOs,
72–73

Rawls, J., 108